INSULIN PUMPS
AND CONTINUOUS
GLUCOSE MONITORING

A USER'S GUIDE TO EFFECTIVE
DIABETES MANAGEMENT

BY FRANCINE R. KAUFMAN, MD

WITH EMILY WESTFALL

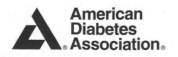

American
Diabetes
Association.

Director, Book Publishing, Abe Ogden; *Managing Editor,* Greg Guthrie; *Acquisitions Editor,* Victor Van Beuren; *Editor,* Greg Guthrie; *Production Manager,* Melissa Sprott; *Composition,* Naylor Design, Inc.; *Cover Design,* Vis-à-vis Creative Concepts, Inc.; *Illustrators,* KTB Studios, LLC, and Jeff Johnston; *Printer,* Versa Press.

Printed in the United States of America
1 3 5 7 9 10 8 6 4 2

The suggestions and information contained in this publication are generally consistent with the *Clinical Practice Recommendations* and other policies of the American Diabetes Association, but they do not represent the policy or position of the Association or any of its boards or committees. Reasonable steps have been taken to ensure the accuracy of the information presented. However, the American Diabetes Association cannot ensure the safety or efficacy of any product or service described in this publication. Individuals are advised to consult a physician or other appropriate health care professional before undertaking any diet or exercise program or taking any medication referred to in this publication. Professionals must use and apply their own professional judgment, experience, and training and should not rely solely on the information contained in this publication before prescribing any diet, exercise, or medication. The American Diabetes Association—its officers, directors, employees, volunteers, and members—assumes no responsibility or liability for personal or other injury, loss, or damage that may result from the suggestions or information in this publication.

∞ The paper in this publication meets the requirements of the ANSI Standard Z39.48-1992 (permanence of paper).

ADA titles may be purchased for business or promotional use or for special sales. To purchase more than 50 copies of this book at a discount, or for custom editions of this book with your logo, contact the American Diabetes Association at the address below, at booksales@diabetes.org, or by calling 703-299-2046.

American Diabetes Association
1701 North Beauregard Street
Alexandria, Virginia 22311

DOI: 10.2337/9781580404617

Library of Congress Cataloging-in-Publication Data
Kaufman, Francine Ratner.
  Insulin pumps and continuous glucose monitoring / Francine R. Kaufman, with Emily Westfall. — 1st ed.
     p. cm.
  Includes bibliographical references and index.
  ISBN 978-1-58040-461-7 (alk. paper)
  1. Insulin pumps. 2. Diabetes—Treatment. 3. Insulin—Therapeutic use. 4. Blood sugar monitoring. 5. Patient education. I. Westfall, Emily. II. American Diabetes Association. III. Title.
  RC661.I63K38 2012
  616.4'62061—dc23

                                                                    2011050394

CONTENTS

ACKNOWLEDGMENTS

I would like to acknowledge the contribution that Dr. Harry Keen made to the field of insulin pump therapy. Harry gave birth to the notion and was visionary in realizing what it could do to improve the lives of those dependent on exogenous insulin treatment. I would also like to acknowledge all that Dr. John Pickup has done to help bring pump therapy to life.

I would like to thank Talia Rabb, who helped me conceive of how to frame this book. I would also like to thank Kelly Joy, Linda Burkett, Kathy Beaver, and Susan Bristol. Their advice and editing were invaluable.

I met Emily Westfall by serendipity on a plane. During that brief encounter, I was so impressed (and in need of help with organizing this book) that I asked her if she wanted to assist me. She was an amazing collaborator, and I am grateful she sat next to me and said yes to my request.

As always, my inspiration comes from my patients and their families, along with my husband, Neal Kaufman, MD, and my own children.

INTRODUCTION

I remember the first insulin pump I used with my patients in the early 1980s. It was jokingly referred to as the "big blue brick," and it weighed several pounds. The insulin-filled syringe was on the outside of the pump, the pump used a butterfly needle (the needle commonly used for intravenous delivery of medications) placed in the subcutaneous tissue, and, for the most part, it could only be used in the hospital setting. I remember feeling that this was a great advance for my patients, and I appreciated that they benefited from the continuous delivery of basal insulin and from the intermittent boluses that were given to match their food intake and to correct an abnormal blood glucose level when indicated. When I reflect back, I realize we have come a long way over the ensuing 30 years. We have witnessed incredible advances in the understanding of what happens to the cells of the body as the result of the diabetes process. We have seen tremendous breakthroughs in diabetes drug discovery, including the development of insulin analogs, and rapid advances in glucose monitoring technology. We have determined better ways to deliver diabetes education and support, and we continue to combat discrimination against people with diabetes. And most importantly for this book, today we have insulin pumps that are small, fast, and smart, and we have continuous glucose monitors (CGMs). CGMs can give information in real time to help with diabetes management decisions. With some devices, the pump and the CGM work together in a single system.

When I diagnose someone with diabetes, I feel as if I start him or her on a new, different life's journey. To succeed on that journey, one must effectively manage diabetes so that the maximal amount of time is spent with glucose levels in the target range, and the minimum amount of time in the low or high range. To accomplish this, people with diabetes, and their parents or caregivers, must track glucose levels to be able to deliver insulin in a manner that closely resembles how the body produces and uses its own insulin. Often the best way to achieve this is to use an insulin pump. And this may be accompanied by using a CGM. These technologies—although not really that much more complicated than your smartphone, computer, or DVD—do require basic understanding, training, and follow-up adjustment if they are going to be helpful in improving diabetes outcomes. The purpose of this book is to give you practical tips, including the knowledge and the skills to maximize insulin pump therapy and continuous glucose monitoring, if that is what you and your health care provider decide is best for you or your child. The goal is to enable you to make your journey through life with diabetes as successful as possible.

SECTION 1: THE BASICS

The goal of section 1 is to review the basic physiology of glucose control and what occurs when someone has diabetes. To understand what you are striving for, you must also be aware of glucose and A1C targets. The central principles of how diabetes is now managed are supported by a series of important research studies. The critical ones, such as the Diabetes Control and Complications Trial (DCCT) and important research studies concerning insulin pump therapy, are reviewed so that you understand the evidence surrounding the recommendations for meticulous diabetes control.

The insulin pump is a small mechanical device worn by someone who has diabetes and who is treated with insulin. The insulin pump helps facilitate diabetes control and lifestyle flexibility. Insulin enters the body from the pump after flowing down the tubing into a small cannula, which is a soft tube, or through a small needle placed under the skin. Newer pumps don't even use tubing. The insulin regimen used by insulin pumps is called basal-bolus therapy, and the benefits of basal-bolus therapy will be outlined. In addition, you'll see how you can balance insulin administration, food, and activity with greater ease while using an insulin pump.

SECTION 2: THE NITTY-GRITTY

Section 2 gets into the practical aspects of insulin pump therapy. The components and features of the pump are described, emphasizing the pump's bolus calculator. Sections on both basal and bolus insulin delivery cover all aspects: from how to determine your initial pump settings to how to adjust settings over time. Because food is a critical element in diabetes management, there is a detailed discussion of carbohydrates, understanding how to read food labels, and ways to assess your portions. One of the true challenges in diabetes management is adjusting insulin and carbohydrate intake for planned and unplanned physical activity. An in-depth review of principles to manage exercise are given in this section.

To succeed with insulin pump therapy, it is critical to understand infusion sets, know how infusion sets differ, and what you need to consider in making the decision about which set you want to use. Although diabetes management can be challenging when you are at home, feeling well, and following your standard routine, special circumstances can make diabetes management more challenging. Situations like illness, traveling (particularly across time zones), or going off to school or college can affect glucose control. Understanding how to adjust your regimen and what do to with your glucose numbers is reviewed in this section.

SECTION 3: ADJUSTING TO INSULIN PUMP THERAPY

Section 3 covers the developmental capabilities of children with regard to managing pumps. You should have realistic expectations of what your child can do with his or her increasing self-management skills. If you don't know what is reasonable, then you might push or hold back your child in the quest for independence.

When you begin pump therapy, it is like starting all over again. You have to check glucose levels more often, wake up in the night, assess and adjust, and think about diabetes all of the time. This can cause stress in and of itself. Deciding whom to tell about your pump, what it means to be attached to a device, and how your body image might be affected are critical issues in accepting—and ultimately succeeding with—pump therapy.

SECTION 4: CONTINUOUS GLUCOSE MONITORING AND PUMPS

There is increasing evidence of the benefits of continuous glucose monitoring. Having a glucose value displayed continuously and the ability to see trends in glucose levels can improve glucose control and help you avoid serious highs and lows. However, continuous glucose monitoring involves adding another device to your self-care toolbox and learning how to use the additional information that comes from it.

The goal of this section is to give you the information you need to start and succeed with continuous glucose monitoring. How the devices work, what the graphs and numbers mean, and how to integrate this new tool into your life will be discussed.

SECTION 5: A LOOK INTO THE FUTURE

Section 5 will give you a glimpse into the future. There is no doubt that the companies involved in diabetes technology, the diabetes associations—including the Juvenile Diabetes Research Foundation (JDRF), the Helmsley Trust, and the American Diabetes Association (ADA)—and many diabetes researchers are interested in seeing the "artificial pancreas" developed to benefit people with diabetes. The goal of the artificial pancreas is to deliver insulin automatically, almost minute to minute, in response to the glucose levels obtained in real time by the glucose sensor—just like the human pancreas does. Achieving this, however, requires a series of algorithms—mathematical equations that take into account a number of things, such as the glucose level at the time, the immediately prior glucose levels, and the rate of change of the glucose value, as well as how much insulin has already been delivered, and insulin sensitivity, to name a few. Ideally, the end result is near-perfect control of glucose levels without much human intervention. The dream of the artificial pancreas will become a reality through incremental steps that will make insulin pumps more automatic in their operation. We already have pumps that automatically suspend insulin delivery for actual hypoglycemia. In the near future, we may see pumps suspend insulin for predicted hypoglycemia, give an automatic bolus for sustained high glucose levels, or completely control insulin delivery during sleep. The future is bright, and sharing its promise with you will conclude the book.

The goal of this book is to help you understand why you or your child might want to use an insulin pump and a CGM, to give you the skills to use them, and to help optimize your or your child's journey with diabetes. Insulin pumps and CGMs may seem overwhelming at the beginning, but trust me, using them can become second nature in no time at all.

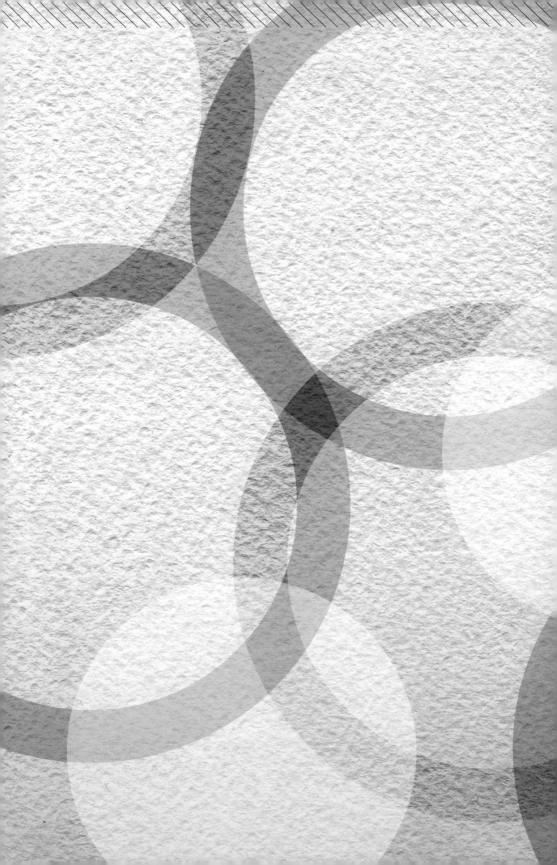

THE BASICS

IN THIS CHAPTER

➡ Remembering Back to Day One

➡ Understanding the Basics about Insulin

➡ Understanding the Transition from Injections to Pumps

➡ Know Your Glucose and A1C Targets

➡ Research Supports Multiple Daily Insulin Injections and Insulin Pump Therapy

CHAPTER 1

WHAT YOU NEED TO KNOW ABOUT DIABETES

REMEMBERING BACK TO DAY ONE

I bet you can remember the day you found out you or your child had diabetes. It is likely that you knew something was wrong for a few days—maybe even weeks—before the diagnosis was made, but you thought it was the flu or a new phase in your life or in your child's development. It is possible you even called your doctor and were told that the problem would go away soon and that there was likely nothing to worry about. Obviously, that wasn't the case.

Some children, teens, and adults are diagnosed with diabetes very early in the process, before they become sick. Some are diagnosed only after they become seriously ill. But most have some, if not all, of the typical signs and symptoms of diabetes: frequent urination, increased thirst, weight loss, and fatigue. These signs and symptoms occur because the pancreas can no longer make enough insulin. Without enough insulin, multiple problems occur with metabolism within the body.

And now remember how remarkable it was just a few days after you were given insulin by injection or through an intravenous infusion (an IV). You were back to your usual self—active, hungry, gaining weight, and learning all about diabetes.

Look back at the first tasks you were asked to do: you had to start to give insulin shots and check blood glucose levels before you had even had a chance to adjust to the fact that you had diabetes. In those first days, you were mostly asked to read, study, and listen to lectures about this disease. You must have felt overwhelmed as it became

I give this Daily Schedule Sheet to my new patients.

DAILY TASKS

Test blood glucose
Determine insulin dose: # grams carb _____ + correction _____
Give insulin
Eat breakfast

Test blood glucose* (This should be 2–2½ hours after last meal)

*If your child would like to eat a snack at this time, you would:
    Determine insulin dose: # grams carb _____ + correction ___
    Give insulin
    Have child eat snack

Test blood glucose
Determine insulin dose: # grams carb _____ + correction _____
Give insulin
Eat lunch

Test blood glucose* (This should be 2–2½ hours after last meal)
*If your child would like to eat a snack at this time, you would:
    Determine insulin dose: # grams carb _____ + correction ___
    Give insulin
    Have child eat snack

apparent you were expected to become an expert, something that took me (and all my health-care-provider friends) years and years to accomplish.

You were likely given a list of things to do and a schedule of when to do them after you were first diagnosed, like in the example above. But essentially, by this time you were aware that every day you need to:

1. Take insulin to be able to metabolize food (mainly carbohydrate) and control the release of glucose from body stores

2. Measure glucose levels throughout the day and night to determine whether insulin doses are working properly

Before 4:30 P.M. call the diabetes team

Test blood glucose
Determine insulin dose: # grams carb _____ + correction _____
Give insulin
Eat dinner

Test blood glucose* (This should be 2–2½ hours after last meal)

*If your child would like to eat a snack at this time, you would:
    Determine insulin dose: # grams carb _____ + correction ___
    Give insulin
    Have child eat snack

At **12:00 A.M. (midnight),** test blood glucose

At **3:00** A.M., test blood glucose

Give basal insulin at _____ daily

3. Eat a healthy and balanced diet, understand the quantity and quality of food, and couple food with taking insulin

4. Be physically active and understand the role of activity in glucose management.

So see how far you have come from those first days? You have come far enough to now consider using an insulin pump and a continuous glucose monitor (CGM)—and to stay committed to doing what you can to optimize your journey with diabetes.

UNDERSTANDING THE BASICS ABOUT INSULIN

In a person who does not have diabetes, the body is designed to control glucose levels in the blood in a very tight range. Although there are fluctuations of glucose levels throughout the day and night, generally glucose levels fall between 70 and 140 mg/dL—highest after eating and lowest after fasting (not eating). Insulin is secreted to keep the glucose that is released from your food or your body's stores moving into your body's cells, where it is used as fuel.

Insulin is secreted in two ways: **1. background (called basal insulin)**, and **2. surges (called bolus insulin)**.

1. **Background (or basal) insulin** controls the glucose levels between meals and overnight. It is mainly acting to help regulate how much glucose is released from the stores in the liver (where it is stored as glycogen). The release of glucose from the liver between meals is critical for providing energy so the body's cells can function. Without enough background or basal insulin, your liver would release too much glucose into the bloodstream and

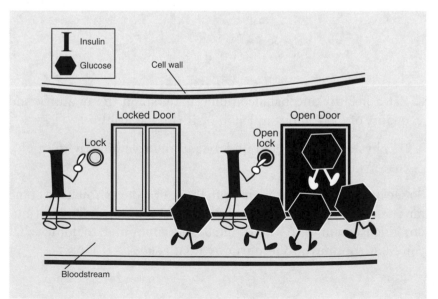

Insulin allows glucose to enter the cells.

your cells would not be able to use it for energy. This could result in very high blood glucose levels. Additionally, without background insulin, the liver will start to produce acidic ketone bodies from the breakdown of fat. Like sugar, these ketone bodies can be measured in the blood and in the urine. As ketones build up in the bloodstream, there is the risk of developing diabetic ketoacidosis (known as DKA). This is potentially a very dangerous condition.

2. **Surge insulin (or bolus)** occurs at mealtime. As glucose levels rise from meals, the pancreas responds with a large increase in insulin release, so the glucose can be used by the body's cells. In the human body without diabetes, these surges are very precise: eat more, and more insulin is released; eat less, and less is released.

With diabetes (always in type 1 and sometimes in type 2), the ability to release insulin is lost. Since the discovery of insulin, replacement insulin therapy has evolved into the modern system we have today. The older system used a fixed approach to insulin replacement (though this is still used today). Although you took only one to three shots a day, you had to take injections at set times and in set amounts. You had to eat the same amount of food at the same time every day, and you had to exercise at the same time every day.

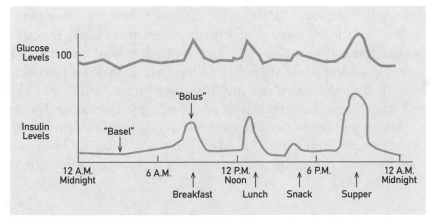

24-hour insulin and glucose profile in a person without diabetes.

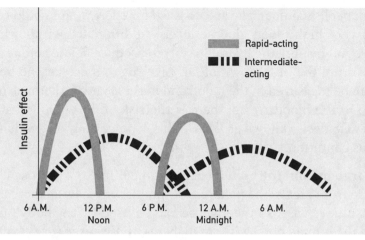

Two shots: a combination of intermediate- and rapid-acting insulins.

This figure shows one way to implement the fixed approach. The person with diabetes takes two shots a day. Each shot is a combination of intermediate- and rapid-acting insulin. As you can see, this approach is not very flexible. For example, if you eat dinner before 6:00 P.M., you won't have a bolus to cover the blood glucose rise. You could take your mixed shot earlier to cover the meal, but then you might not have any insulin in your system overnight. If you eat early but take your shot at the regular time, then you could have a high that is untreated.

With this old way, keeping glucose in the target range was very difficult. And there was no flexibility in life. Essentially, your life had to fit into the diabetes regimen. The diabetes regimen controlled you.

The newer way to treat diabetes is with flexible regimens: multiple daily injections (MDI) or insulin pump therapy. These newer, flexible systems mimic the way the pancreas normally produces and releases insulin. MDI mimics background insulin and surges of insulin. It allows you to deliver insulin in doses to match your food intake and gives you flexibility in how much you eat and when you eat it. You can be active when you want, and with an insulin pump you can decrease basal insulin in order to avoid hypoglycemia. You can sleep when you want, wake up late, and travel around the globe with the flexibility to change from one day to the next.

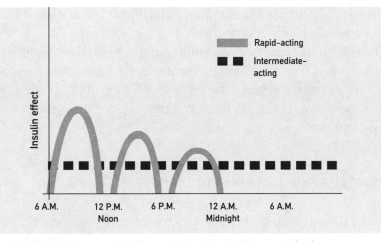

How an MDI regimen covers insulin requirements over the course of a day.

This figure shows how MDI covers insulin requirements over a 24-hour period. Because your basal and bolus insulins aren't tied together, you can take the bolus shot when you need it, giving you more flexibility in your lifestyle.

UNDERSTANDING THE TRANSITION FROM INJECTIONS TO PUMPS

You are likely taking multiple injections of insulin every day—possibly two or three injections (perhaps using NPH insulin)—but you are most likely on MDI. With MDI, you use rapid-acting insulin and long-acting or basal insulin. These two different kinds of insulins have different jobs, but both work to keep your glucose in the target range.

Basal insulin is given as one or two shots each day, and it activates slowly after injection. This means that some amount of insulin will always be present in the blood. The blood can then bring insulin to the cells throughout the body, and glucose can then enter the cells, where it is converted into energy. In the liver, insulin helps regulate the slow release of stored glucose to meet the energy needs of the body's cells between meals and during the night.

Bolus insulin is given as rapid-acting insulin. It is activated much faster after injection and brings the large amount of glucose from your meals into your body's cells. There, glucose can be used right away for energy or stored for later use. Boluses with rapid-acting insulin can also be used to decrease a high blood glucose level. These doses are called correction boluses.

The difference between an insulin pump and MDI is that an insulin pump just uses rapid-acting insulin to do both jobs. The basal rates on the pump replace the basal insulin injection in MDI, and boluses given at meals and for correction replace the mealtime and correction shots.

KNOW YOUR GLUCOSE AND A1C TARGETS

What is the ultimate goal of diabetes treatment? To effectively manage diabetes day to day, so that glucose levels are in the right range—known as the target range—as much as possible to avoid highs and lows. Keeping glucose levels in the target range minimizes your risk of the short- and long-term complications. The target range for glucose is different at different times of the day. For example, in the morning when you haven't eaten for several hours (fasting), your target will be lower than it is after meals, when blood glucose is highest.

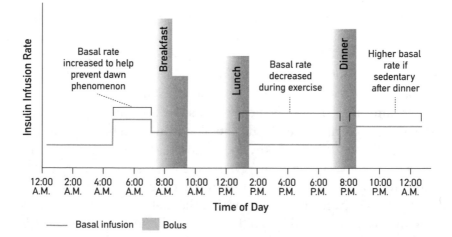

When you use an insulin pump, your basal rate and boluses are customized to more closely mimic how the body releases its own insulin. Both the basal infusion and the boluses are made with rapid-acting insulin.

Overnight, when you are sleeping, your target may be higher than the fasting range to protect you from hypoglycemia.

The American Diabetes Association (ADA) has established general target ranges for glucose levels throughout the day for different age groups. Generally speaking, younger children have higher targets for their glucose levels. In addition, there are a number of conditions that might lead the diabetes team to suggest higher targets, such as having repeated low blood glucose (hypoglycemia), being unaware of the symptoms of hypoglycemia (referred to as hypoglycemia unawareness), or having diabetes complications. You should discuss this with your diabetes team and find out what your target range glucose levels should be throughout the day and night.

Similarly, you should be aware of the target range for your A1C test. A1C measures the percentage (%) of your hemoglobin (a protein in red blood cells) molecules that have glucose attached to them. The higher your average glucose levels day after day, the higher your A1C. It gives you a good picture of what your blood glucose levels have been in general over a longer amount of time. A1C should be measured every three to four months, and you should know what your level is each time it is taken. A1C is often referred to as the diabetes report card. By seeing if your A1C is in the target range set by your diabetes team, you can know if your diabetes control is optimal.

RESEARCH SUPPORTS MDI AND INSULIN PUMP THERAPY

There have been a lot of research studies in the fields of MDI and insulin pump therapy, and many of them have shown that there are potential benefits in diabetes care. Here are some studies that have helped us better understand how to manage diabetes and how MDI and particularly insulin pump therapy can be a useful tool.

The Diabetes Control and Complications Trial (DCCT)

Before the mid-1990s, someone with type 1 diabetes would take one (maybe two or, rarely, three) insulin injections per day. Back then,

Blood Glucose Targets for Children, Teens, and Adults

Age	Goal for plasma blood glucose range (mg/dL)		A1C (%)
	Before meals	Bedtime/overnight	
Toddlers and preschoolers (<6 years)	100–180	110–200	7.5–8.5
School age (6–12 years)	90–180	100–180	<8
Adolescents (13–19 years)	90–130	90–150	<7.5
Adults	80–130	90–150	<7.0

This is adapted from the article "Care of Children and Adolescents with Type 1 Diabetes: A statement of the American Diabetes Association," by Janet Silverstein, et al., published in *Diabetes Care* 28:186–212, 2010.

regular, NPH, lente, and ultralente insulins were in use. Except for NPH and regular, these other insulin preparations are not available today. Insulin doses weren't adjusted from one day to the next, which meant that people had to follow a strict eating plan and physical activity regimen. That meant you couldn't skip breakfast, you couldn't delay having lunch, and if you routinely had a snack in the afternoon, you had to eat one even if you weren't hungry! Although you might have taken fewer shots, the trade-off in having a fixed diet and activity pattern wasn't worth it—and more importantly, this regimen led to inadequate diabetes control.

The Diabetes Control and Complications Trial (known as the DCCT) was a nine-year study. When the results were reported in 1993, the concept of how diabetes should be managed was changed forever. The investigators proved that tighter glucose control using MDI (three or more shots per day) or insulin pump therapy was better than conventional therapy at lowering A1C and reducing the risks of developing diabetes complications.

The DCCT conclusively showed that blood glucose control matters. Although the youngest participants in the DCCT were 13 years old when they entered the study, the overall results of the DCCT have been generalized to all of type 1 diabetes: effective blood glucose control is the most effective way to reduce the long-term complications of diabetes.

Over 1,400 people with type 1 diabetes took part in the study. They were divided among two groups: one for intensive management and the other for conventional therapy (the way diabetes used to be managed). The intensive group used MDI (three or more shots per day) or an insulin pump. This group also received a great deal of support from the study teams. At the end of the DCCT, the people who used MDI had an average A1C level of 7.4%. Those receiving conventional therapy took one or two shots a day, and did not have blood glucose targets or a lot of support from the study teams. Their average A1C levels were 9.1%. Nine years later, those in the intensive group had fewer severe eye, kidney, and nerve problems than those in the conventional group. This was a stunning discovery. However, the other lesson from the DCCT was that lowering A1C levels increases the risk of hypoglycemia.

Epidemiology of Diabetes Interventions and Complications (EDIC)

After the DCCT concluded in 1993, a follow-up study began, and it is still running today. The study is called Epidemiology of Diabetes Interventions and Complications (EDIC), and almost all of the DCCT participants entered into it (but they did return to their previous health care teams, not the study teams). By 2009, those who had been in the intensive group had lower rates of eye disease, kidney disease, and cardiovascular disease when compared with those in the conventional group. Although the people in the intensive group did see an increase in their average A1C levels over this period, there was still convincing evidence that intensive management and improved A1C levels provide noticeable health benefits,

LESSONS FROM DCCT AND EDIC

After 30 years of diabetes, fewer than 1% of participants in the intensive group had become blind, required kidney replacement, or had an amputation because of diabetes.

even if the therapy was provided years before. That is why considering an insulin pump to manage your diabetes makes sense.

Other Studies and Guidelines

Many studies have evaluated insulin pump therapy. Although none have had the scientific rigor of the DCCT, overall they show that insulin pump therapy decreases A1C, and now it has also been shown to reduce rates of hypoglycemia. These studies have been done across age groups, for different conditions (such as pregnancy or severe hypoglycemia), and in many places around the globe. There have been 11 studies that compared insulin pumps to MDI, and across all of them, A1C was approximately 0.5% lower in those using insulin pumps. Regardless of who is using the insulin pump, the studies have shown an overwhelmingly positive benefit.

Studies with Sensors and Sensor-Augmented Pumps

A CGM is a device that can give information in real time to help with diabetes management decisions. With some devices, the pump and the CGM work together in a single system. The expanded availability and use of CGMs can be partially credited to clinical research into this new device. Some of the studies looked at the use of insulin pump therapy integrated with a CGM. This type of therapy is often called sensor-augmented pump therapy, or SAPT. Other studies looked at the benefits of individuals using a CGM either with an insulin pump or with MDI.

The Juvenile Diabetes Research Foundation (JDRF) sponsored one of the largest studies ever done on CGMs. The study included 322 adults and children who were receiving intensive therapy for type 1 diabetes (either with an insulin pump or MDI). After six months, adults showed improved blood glucose control. A subset of children and adults whose A1C values were less than 7.0% at the beginning of the study was also analyzed. In this group of individuals, low blood glucose (hypoglycemia) was less frequent, time spent out of the target blood glucose range was shorter, and average A1C levels were still excellent. The benefits of CGM go beyond just the clinical benefits and improved glucose control: the adults and parents of children who used CGM were also pleased with this method of treatment.

In 2010, the results of the STAR 3 study were published in the *New England Journal of Medicine*. The STAR 3 study is the largest study of its kind, and it examined the benefits of SAPT in people with type 1 diabetes comparing it against MDI. The study demonstrated that in both children and adults with inadequately controlled type 1 diabetes, SAPT improved A1C levels. A1C levels were 0.6% lower than those in the MDI group. Also, a greater number of individuals reached their A1C target levels.

Once the STAR 3 study was completed, the patients receiving MDI in the first year of the study were placed on SAPT for six months. They were compared with the people who received SAPT during the first year of the study and who continued on SAPT for the same six-month period. There was a significant and sustained decrease in A1C levels in the children and adults who went from MDI to SAPT for the final six months of the study.

One of the most important lessons we've learned from all of the clinical studies done with SAPT is that the biggest treatment benefit is seen in those individuals who use CGM on a consistent and sustained basis. The greatest improvement in blood glucose control was seen in individuals who wore the CGM for more than 60% of the time. This was true for children, adolescents, and adults.

Guidelines

In 2005, the American Diabetes Association published its guidelines for the management of diabetes in children: "The Care of Children and Adolescents with Type 1 Diabetes." Here are a few of the key items from those guidelines:

- Insulin pump use is widespread in children with diabetes.

- There is no correct age at which to initiate insulin pump therapy, so treatment plans should consider the needs of the patient as well as those of the family to determine who is an appropriate candidate for an insulin pump and when he or she should begin pump therapy.

- The support of adults at home and at school is essential for the child's success with all diabetes management, but especially with pump therapy.

Other medical associations have published recommendations. The International Society for Pediatric and Adolescent Diabetes published theirs in 2009. That guideline explains that insulin pump therapy is the best way to imitate how a human body without diabetes provides insulin. The American Association of Clinical Endocrinologists has a consensus statement that discusses the broad groups of patients with type 1 and type 2 diabetes who may benefit from insulin pump therapy.

CHAPTER REVIEW

➡ Appreciate how far you have come since your original diagnosis. You have learned so much about diabetes management, the tasks you need to perform, and ways to better control your glucose levels.

➡ The concepts of basal and bolus insulin delivery are the keys to pump therapy. Either method can be adjusted throughout the day and night to improve glucose control.

➡ Transitioning from MDI to pump therapy means you go from taking two (or maybe even more) kinds of insulin to one—only rapid-acting insulin.

➡ You should know your blood glucose and A1C targets. You adjust your insulin doses, food intake, and activity levels to reach your glucose targets throughout the day and night. At your diabetes visits, find out your A1C so you can know if you have achieved your goal.

➡ There is a lot of evidence from scientific studies that shows the benefits of insulin pump therapy. Pumps reduce hypoglycemia, improve A1C levels, improve quality of life, and reduce daily insulin dosages. CGM has the ability to further improve diabetes care, particularly when used most of the time.

CHAPTER 2

AN OVERVIEW OF INSULIN PUMPS

WHAT EXACTLY IS AN INSULIN PUMP?

Simply put, an insulin pump is a device to deliver insulin. It is a small mechanical device that is worn externally. It is prescribed by your physician, and your diabetes team will determine your starting doses. You will need to learn how to program the pump, and then you will be responsible for telling it how much insulin to give you. You program it to provide both basal (the background insulin) and bolus insulin (for meals and correction doses). A computer in the pump regulates the flow of insulin into the body. An insulin pump eliminates the use of daily injections and uses only rapid-acting insulin both for the basal rates and for boluses.

Durable Pumps and Patch Pumps

Durable insulin pumps are about the size of a deck of cards and can come in a variety of types and colors. Most pumps are connected to the body by tubing. This tubing runs from a reservoir filled with insulin in the pump to an infusion set, which is secured to your body. The infusion set is made up of a small 6–9 mm (less than 1/2 inch) soft plastic cannula that is inserted under the skin. It is inserted by a needle, which is then removed. The cannula can also be a very small steel needle that is easily inserted under the skin. The computer in the pump controls a motor that that dispenses the insulin in tiny amounts. The insulin flows from the reservoir into the tubing and then through the cannula into the tissue under the skin. There is a display screen on the pump, and buttons to program insulin delivery.

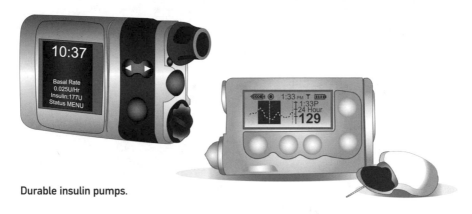

Durable insulin pumps.

Patch pumps are attached directly to the body. They do not have an infusion set or tubing. The insulin reservoir is inside the patch, and you fill the reservoir before placing the patch on your body. There is a needle that places a small cannula under the skin, and this needle then retracts back, so it is no longer in the body. These pumps have a separate controller that communicates with the motor in the patch to control insulin release. There is no display screen on the patch; all interactions are made through the controller, which wirelessly transmits the commands to the patch pump.

Those are just the basics. As we go on, you will learn more about what pumps can do, how they work, and what other features pumps have.

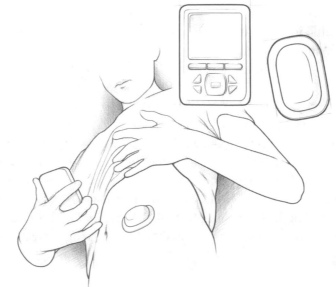

Patch pump.

THE ADVANTAGES OF PUMPS

Insulin pumps can be used to effectively manage your diabetes. They can help you achieve your blood glucose and A1C targets. They give you flexibility. Many people feel as if their quality of life has been enhanced by insulin pump therapy, and they feel like they are more in control. Let's go over what else insulin pumps offer.

Multiple Basal Rates

Multiple basal rates can be used to avoid high and low glucose levels. Many people have specific patterns that can be addressed by changing their basal rates throughout the day and night. For example, if you have the dawn phenomenon (high blood glucose in the morning), then increasing the basal insulin rates at 3:00 A.M. may help you avoid it. If you go to the gym in the afternoon, basal rates can be decreased to avoid hypoglycemia. Adjustable rates can also be helpful if you have hypoglycemia unawareness (you don't recognize the signs of low blood glucose), gastroparesis (a digestive disorder), or an unpredictable lifestyle.

Temporary Basal Rates

Pumps allow you to temporarily change basal insulin delivery. You can either increase or decrease it. This helps when you are ill (when you are not eating and are at risk for hypoglycemia), have high blood glucose from stress, have exercised more than usual, or are traveling across time zones. In addition, you can use temporary basal rates to help treat highs and lows as they occur.

Multiple Basal Patterns

You can have more than one 24-hour basal pattern from which to select. For example, when insulin sensitivity changes with menstruation (for women), you can program a separate 24-hour basal pattern that increases basal delivery all day long. You can have separate 24-hour basal patterns for weekdays and weekends (when you want to sleep in), for traveling, or for summer vacation.

Avoidance of Long-Acting and Intermediate-Acting Insulin

You use only rapid-acting insulin in the pump. If you use injections, you use long-acting or intermediate-acting insulin in addition to rapid-acting insulin. In an ideal world, long-acting insulin would be absorbed evenly over many hours, without any peak effect. Similarly, intermediate-acting insulin (or NPH insulin) has peaks that are supposed to be timed to meals. But neither of these insulins is completely predictably absorbed from one day to the next. This variation in insulin absorption may contribute to unexplained high and low glucose levels that can be seen with injection treatments; these fluctuations in blood glucose levels are less frequent with insulin pump therapy.

Precision in Insulin Delivery

Pumps deliver insulin with precision, particularly when compared with insulin injections. Insulin pumps can deliver very small amounts of insulin, as low as 0.025 unit. By contrast, the lowest a syringe can deliver accurately is 0.5 unit.

Dosing for Food Intake

Choosing the right dose of insulin for a meal is a huge challenge, particularly if you eat out a lot, like to snack, or aren't sure what's in your foods. With a pump, you can take multiple boluses by pressing a few buttons, in case you eat more than you planned. You can take one bolus to start with and then take another if you realize the portion you ate was more than you had intended. (Just be careful that you don't take too many boluses.) An insulin pump also makes it much easier to take your dose before you begin to eat, which can be difficult when you are in public and have to give yourself a shot.

Bolus Calculators

Most insulin pumps have bolus calculators that help determine how much insulin is needed for food and for correcting hyperglycemia. By programming your insulin-to-carbohydrate ratio and correction factor (how much insulin you need to bring high glucose down to the intended range) into the pump, the bolus calculator will do the math and provide you with an estimate of how much insulin you need to give.

Dosing to Correct Hyperglycemia

Because the pump already has your programmed insulin correction factor, it is easier to take a bolus to correct a high glucose level. Once the glucose level is entered into the pump, the pump will calculate how much insulin is needed. With the push of a few buttons, treatment for hyperglycemia is on the way.

Weight Management

Some people can improve their weight, if they need to do so, with an insulin pump. This can occur if the person experiences less hypoglycemia and no longer needs to consume extra carbohydrate to treat it.

Child Safety Features

Many insulin pumps have features that protect children from accidentally delivering extra insulin or changing pump settings.

Summing Up the Advantages

You can eat when you want, be active when you choose, wake up when you want, take multiple boluses, have options for basal infusion rates, and get help with insulin dose calculations. This should lead to better diabetes control, more glucose levels within your target range with fewer highs and lows, better A1C, and a better journey with diabetes.

THE DISADVANTAGES OF PUMPS

Even though there are many advantages to insulin pump therapy, there are some disadvantages. Understanding them is important, because deciding to go on insulin pump therapy should be a carefully considered decision.

Risk of Diabetic Ketoacidosis (DKA)

Because the pump only uses rapid-acting insulin, if there is an unexpected or accidental interruption of insulin delivery, there may not be enough insulin in the bloodstream to stop the liver from releasing glucose and producing ketones. This can rapidly progress to DKA, which is a serious medical condition. By closely monitoring glucose levels, checking for ketones, and dosing insulin to bring glucose and ketone levels down, DKA can be avoided. You can find out more about DKA in chapter 9.

Being Attached

Some people feel apprehensive about wearing an insulin pump all day, every day, and about being attached to a device, no matter how small it is. This was probably a bigger issue before we all became comfortable having cell phones with us 24/7. The insulin pump will be attached to you, and for some people that is a constant reminder that they have diabetes. Try to view the insulin pump as a key to good control and a healthy, more normal life.

Privacy

People can see your insulin pump, unless you conceal it. The pump will make it difficult to hide the fact that you have diabetes. If you are reluctant to let people know about your diabetes, then this is something to consider before starting insulin pump therapy.

Skin Issues

The infusion set and the tape can irritate the skin. To use a pump, you may have to try different combinations of tape and skin treatments until you find what works for you. If you use the same site for the infusion set repeatedly, you can get scar tissue and an increase in fatty tissue buildup (called lipohypertrophy).

Infusion Set Issues

The probability of your infusion set falling out or being jarred from the site can be minimized with good habits. Using appropriate taping techniques and changing your infusion set regularly can help avert problems. To be safe, you need to keep extra pump supplies with you at school or work, and have an insulin pen or syringe available so you never have to compromise your safety and health.

Missing Boluses

Some people forget to bolus with meals or to correct hyperglycemia. If you regularly miss or skip taking a bolus for food, then your A1C will increase. The good news is that many pumps have alarms that you can set to remind you to test or take a bolus at certain times; an example might be to set a bolus alarm to remind you at lunchtime to check your glucose and take your bolus insulin. You can also set the alarm on your phone or watch to remind you about boluses.

Weight Gain

Some people gain weight due to the ease of dosing insulin. But the pump doesn't add excess calories to your meal plan—only you can do that. Remember your meal plan, and schedule a meeting with a registered dietitian if you're having trouble following your healthy eating plan.

Cost

The insulin pump itself, plus the supplies (e.g., infusion sets, insulin reservoirs, tapes), have a cost. Most insurance companies cover insulin pump therapy, minus your deductible. It is important for you to find out what you will have to pay out of pocket for insulin pump therapy before you make the transition.

Summing Up the Disadvantages

These disadvantages usually become less significant as time passes and as you become more familiar with the pump. As your knowledge and experiences grow, you will be able to adapt to the pump and make it work for you. Insulin pumps can be a great tool for diabetes management and can mean better glucose control and fewer complications.

WHAT MAKES YOU A GOOD PUMP CANDIDATE?

Before anyone can take on an insulin pump, he or she needs to understand what the pump can do and how it works, be realistic about his or her capabilities, and know a good deal about diabetes management. Your diabetes team may be very enthusiastic about pump therapy for you, but are you ready for it? What do you need to do to be considered ready for an insulin pump?

- **Realistic expectations.** The pump is not an artificial pancreas. It doesn't cure diabetes. It cannot correct anything on its own. This is true even if you have a sensor and use CGM. You must be committed to being very active in your diabetes—and pump—management. Successful management takes time, good habits, dedication, hard work, and commitment.

- **No coercion.** No one should be forced to get an insulin pump, including young children. Although a pump can motivate someone to participate in his or her diabetes management, this cannot be the primary reason to get a child or teen an insulin pump.

- **Participation of others.** No one can manage diabetes alone. Children, teens, and young adults need someone—a family member or a friend—who understands diabetes, insulin pumps, and diabetes emergencies.

- **Sufficient diabetes knowledge.** To succeed with pump therapy, it is important to understand the following concepts: basal/bolus therapy, your diabetes meal plan, carbohydrate counting, avoiding and treating hyperglycemia, and sick-day management. Gaining skills and knowledge should be your goal.

- **Awareness of financial responsibilities.** Find out exactly what your insurance will cover and what you will have to pay out of pocket. This is vital information.

- **Sufficient glucose monitoring.** The only way to effectively use an insulin pump is to check your glucose frequently and take action based on the glucose levels. Many health care providers and insurance carriers require proof of four or more glucose checks a day for at least 60 days before they will authorize you to get a pump. Without adequate glucose monitoring, pump therapy is less likely to be successful.

GETTING AN INSULIN PUMP

If you are ready for an insulin pump and are confident that you meet the requirements listed above, then you'll need to work with your diabetes team to determine which pump you should get.

Which Pump?

Different companies make different pumps. Although these different pumps are fundamentally similar, each individual pump has its own distinguishing features. Likewise, different pump manufacturers provide different services. Discuss the available options with your diabetes team, research them on the Internet, read the product brochures, talk to people who use pumps, and learn as much as possible. Decide what features or services are important to you. Once you have made your choice, work with your diabetes team, the insulin pump company, and a pump trainer to make your new journey successful and enjoyable.

When to Start Pump Therapy

There is no right or wrong time to start insulin pump therapy. It is becoming more common for people to begin pump therapy early in the course of their diabetes, while others wait for some time. Some decide to get an insulin pump only after they have had a problem, like severe hypoglycemia, or a complication. Sometimes the diabetes team is pushing for pump therapy; other times, team members are reluctant. Some health care providers are more willing to use pumps, and others have very strict criteria for who they think is a good candidate.

At the present time, pump therapy is usually considered to be the next step after MDI. If your diabetes center uses MDI at the time of the diagnosis of diabetes, it might only take weeks or months to

IF YOU'RE READY FOR AN INSULIN PUMP, HERE'S WHAT'S NEXT...

Your physician has to prescribe the insulin pump, and your insurance company will have to review and approve the claim. Your pump will be shipped to you or your health care professional. You will be given instructions on how to start learning about your new device.

switch to a pump. If your diabetes center starts people on one to three shots per day in a fixed regimen, then you likely have to go to MDI and then to a pump. This could take months or years.

Is there an advantage to starting insulin pump therapy earlier rather than later? Perhaps, but we don't really know for sure. However, studies are underway to determine if more intensive management at diagnosis is beneficial.

Pump Training

Before you have your in-person pump training, do some research. Most companies have some easy online learning that will help you become familiar with how your pump operates. Your pump trainer will be certified in all of the features of your insulin pump and will verify that you know how to operate it. You will go through all the steps of setting up the pump, filling the reservoir, priming and inserting your infusion set, and practicing as many times as you need until you are comfortable and confident with the pump. There are online tools, instructional videos, and booklets to give you further guidance after training.

Data Management with Computer Programs

You can upload the information stored in your insulin pump to a computer program, which is either supplied by the manufacturer of your pump or available from another company. The program will allow you to store and upload information, such as number of insulin doses delivered, pump settings, glucose values, carbohydrates consumed, infusion set changes, pump suspends, and more. These data management programs then display data in pie charts, tables, graphs, and percentages above and below target range. The ability to transfer this data and analyze it with the software can help you improve your diabetes care by making it easier to detect trends and patterns that may require attention.

CHAPTER REVIEW

➡ An insulin pump is a small machine that continuously delivers insulin. Pumps come in two varieties: durable and patch.

➡ There are many advantages to insulin pump therapy. The advantages of delivering basal insulin with a pump include multiple basal rates, temporary basal rates, multiple basal patterns, and precise insulin delivery. Boluses can be given to cover food, to correct an elevated glucose level, or both. This gives you flexibility.

➡ The disadvantages include the risk of DKA, the issues of being attached to a device that reminds you about diabetes and might be visible to others, issues with your skin and with infusion sets, missed boluses because diabetes management becomes more automatic, and cost.

➡ Pump users should have these qualities: realistic expectations, ability to participate with others in their diabetes care, sufficient diabetes knowledge, willingness to monitor glucose effectively, desire to use an insulin pump, and an understanding of the costs of the device.

➡ You need to decide which pump to use, and getting properly trained is critical.

THE NITTY-GRITTY

CHAPTER 3

HOW DOES MY PUMP WORK?

THE PARTS OF THE PUMP

Although it's only about the size of a deck of cards, an insulin pump is an impressive, complicated device that contains many components and can perform many different functions. There are two kinds of pumps: durable and patch.

Durable pumps are designed to last many years. They are made of a hard plastic case with buttons, a front screen, a battery compartment with a screw on top, and a space for the reservoir that will be filled with insulin. Clips can be attached to the outer surface so you can place the pump on a belt or waistband. There is a sticker on the pump that has some useful information: the serial number, model and type, company phone numbers, and other general information. At the base of the reservoir shaft is a computer-controlled mechanical plunger that can deliver incredibly small amounts of insulin.

Patch pumps are worn directly on the body. The pod component attaches to the body and has the insulin reservoir and motor inside. It is controlled by a separate controller or personal digital assistant (PDA).

Reservoir

The reservoir comes empty. There is a needle attachment that is used to draw insulin from the insulin vial into the reservoir. The needle is detached once the correct amount of insulin is drawn up; the correct amount depends on how much insulin you use in two or three days. The whole reservoir is screw-turned tightly into the chamber in the pump, and the tubing leads away to the infusion set, which is attached to the body. With a patch pump, the reservoir is contained within the pod, which adheres to the skin.

Screen

The pump has a front screen (the patch pump has the screen on the controller). When not in use, front screens generally display the time (some have the date), insulin remaining, and information about battery life. By pushing different buttons on the face of the pump, you can access different functions in the pump's software. The software lets you deliver insulin; set or edit basal rates; set or edit the pump calculator; suspend insulin delivery; review your bolus, basal, and alarm histories; and see the exact amount of insulin remaining in the reservoir.

Software

The software not only lets you know the date and time, it also allows your pump to store tons of information, including weeks' or months' worth of bolus and alarm histories, blood glucose readings, and basal rates. The software allows the pump to consistently deliver the correct amount of basal insulin. It can also calculate the appropriate amount of insulin needed based on a glucose reading and a carb count entered into the system. Some pumps have a large database of food and carb counts. There are also safety features that prevent the user from providing too much or too little insulin in boluses or for the basal rate. Software also allows you to determine how you want to deliver a bolus every time you deliver one.

Pump History and Downloading

The information stored in the pump can be uploaded to a computer and analyzed by software. Generally the pump connects to the computer using a cable or wireless connection, and once the information is transferred from the pump to a computer, the user can look at graphs, pie charts, lists, and other visual information. Many diabetes care providers download information from the pump during clinic visits, or they may ask you to download it at home and bring a printed copy to your appointment. Between visits, you should look at this information and send it to your diabetes team if you need help troubleshooting some problems.

Blood and Interstitial Glucose Monitoring

Most pumps can connect to a blood glucose meter. In addition, it is possible for some of them to connect wirelessly to a continuous glucose monitor (CGM). This means that the glucose meter and sensor can transmit glucose values directly to the pump's screen and memory.

PUMP FUNCTIONS

Insulin Delivery

Pumps deliver basal and bolus rates of insulin. Basal rates are set by the user, with guidance from the diabetes team. Based on individual dosing, mealtime and correction boluses are given.

Suspend

All pumps have the ability to be suspended so that no insulin (basal or bolus) can be administered. A pump can remain suspended indefinitely but will sound an alarm every so often to remind you that you are not receiving insulin. With most pumps, it is easy to suspend insulin delivery in case you have an emergency.

Alarms

Pumps have alarms. Some are functionally important, such as "low battery" or "no delivery" (called an "occlusion" alarm in some pumps). There are alarms that you can set to remind you to test, take insulin, or check for ketones if your glucose is over a certain amount. If you need to, you can review the last 50 or so alarms. Pumps have different options for the way they notify you, such as various beeps or sounds or with vibration. Most pumps will beep or vibrate when a bolus is complete, when you are currently using a temporary basal rate, or when you have a low reservoir or low battery.

Active Insulin or Insulin on Board

After a bolus is given, insulin continues to affect your glucose level for some time. The amount of insulin left in your bloodstream is referred to as "active insulin" or "insulin on board." You can set how long you want the pump to track active insulin, but discuss with your health care team how long you should have the pump track it. Generally, people set the active insulin time to two to five hours (most often, three). The pump calculator keeps track of the amount of insulin that is still active from previous boluses so you do not have boluses overlapping each other and dropping your glucose levels (this is referred to as "insulin stacking").

Maximal Bolus and Basal Rates

You set a maximal rate for both basal and bolus insulin delivery to enhance safety. This prohibits you from accidently taking 20.0 units instead of 2.0, for example.

Pump Bolus Calculators Make Pumps Smart

The pump bolus calculator—which makes pumps smart—calculates how much insulin to give for boluses. It takes into account your insulin-to-carbohydrate ratio (ICR), the insulin sensitivity factor (ISF), the duration of active insulin, and your target glucose range. These values (except active insulin) can be altered by time of day, for example, because your insulin sensitivity and your ICR change over the course of 24 hours. When you first get your pump, your diabetes care team will help you determine these settings. They can be changed at any time (preferably in consultation with your diabetes team) as indicated by the patterns in your glucose control.

To determine the amount of insulin you take for a food bolus, you enter the number of grams of carbohydrate you plan to ingest and your current blood glucose level. Then the pump calculator will determine how much insulin you should take. If your blood glucose is above or below your target range, the bolus calculator will also figure out if you need to add or subtract insulin from the food dose.

However, you can always alter the insulin bolus dose suggested by the pump bolus calculator, giving yourself less or more insulin depending on any number of factors. If you are about to exercise or are not sure you will eat an entire meal, you might want to decrease your bolus from what the calculator suggests. If you have ketones or are sick, you might want to take more. Although it is convenient to have the pump calculator so you don't have to do the calculations yourself, it is important to think before you push the button.

Here's an example. If your blood glucose is 250 mg/dL and you are about to eat 15 grams of carbohydrate for lunch, you would enter those numbers into your bolus calculator (or the blood glucose would be automatically sent from your meter). The calculator suggests an amount of insulin to bring your glucose into your target range and cover your meal. Some pumps will show you the two different amounts, one for food and one for correction, and others will simply lump them together into one suggested bolus without showing a breakdown.

UPLOADING AND RECORD KEEPING

Keeping detailed records of your blood glucose levels, doses of insulin, food intake, and other events (such as exercise, illness, or stress) is important. It is also hard to keep a logbook or a record of all that you do every day. However, when this information is available for review, you are able to spot patterns and trends that may be problematic. In contrast, if you are looking only at your current glucose level, you won't detect these patterns, even if you correct your high glucose nearly every morning and treat a low every afternoon.

By uploading data from your pump to the software, especially when it also includes information from your glucose meter (and a CGM, if you have one), you are able to review up to three months of data. Because the bolus calculator captures the carbohydrate history for meals and breaks out the bolus details so you can see when correction doses were administered, you have the ability to look for trends and patterns. By reviewing these data, you can identify *what* the problems are, why they are occurring, and how they can be fixed.

A Diabetes Meeting

The purpose of a diabetes meeting is to sit down with your diabetes team and review your glucose trends and patterns, your pump (and CGM) settings, and how you are doing with your diabetes regimen. The frequency should be weekly, or less often if there are no issues with your diabetes. The purpose of a diabetes meeting is to identify patterns and trends in your glucose levels, alterations that need to be made in your pump (and CGM) settings, or behaviors that you are looking to improve, such as remembering to bolus, measuring blood glucose levels, using the bolus calculator, and changing infusion sets at least every three days, and more. Set goals, monitor your progress over time, and reward yourself for achieving your goals. After you review your information, discuss it with someone—a friend, spouse, child, parent—and, if needed, with your health care team.

Interpreting Data

There are several ways to look at your pump or meter data. These include a logbook, trend graphs, pie charts, and data tables. The logbook is just a digital version of a handwritten log. Trend graphs, pie charts, and data tables are visual representations of the logbook information that make it easier to spot patterns and trends. The trend graphs and pie charts are colorful visual representations of your glucose numbers, averages, and high/low patterns, whereas the data table contains just numbers and values. Each method of displaying your information can be reviewed to identify specific problems or times of good control.

Logbooks

Logbooks, like the paper ones you were first given when you were diagnosed, are grids containing all of the pertinent information that affects your diabetes. They are either very detailed or they can just display your glucose values at certain times of day (before or after meals).

Trend Graphs

A trend graph is often the first thing that your diabetes team will look at because they easily show many days of data laid over each

Sample Logbook Page.

	Breakfast	Lunch	Dinner	Daily Totals

Legend:
- ▓ >140mg/dL
- ░ <70mg/dL
- 00* Multiple readings (most extreme shown)
- ◯ Manual bolus or bolus with correction
- .... Skipped meal
- <<< Pump rewind
- ^ Suspend

Daily Totals

TUESDAY 8/16/2011	Average (15): 217mg/dL	Carbs: 166g	Insulin: 13.0U Bolus: 64%
WEDNESDAY 8/17/2011	Average (19): 106mg/dL	Carbs: 412g	Insulin: 35.3U Bolus: 63%
THURSDAY 8/18/2011	Average (20): 171mg/dL	Carbs: 190g	Insulin: 30.8U Bolus: 57%
FRIDAY 8/19/2011 <<<	Average (14): 140mg/dL	Carbs: 274g	Insulin: 30.2U Bolus: 57%
SATURDAY 8/20/2011	Average (14): 105mg/dL	Carbs: 246g	Insulin: 30.7U Bolus: 53%
SUNDAY 8/21/2011 <<<	Average (10): 144mg/dL	Carbs: 173g	Insulin: 29.6U Bolus: 52%
MONDAY 8/22/2011	Average (14): 165mg/dL	Carbs: 133g	Insulin: 28.2U Bolus: 47%
TUESDAY 8/23/2011	Average (13): 134mg/dL	Carbs: 296g	Insulin: 42.0U Bolus: 63%
WEDNESDAY 8/24/2011 <<<	Average (13): 141mg/dL	Carbs: 215g	Insulin: 35.6U Bolus: 56%
THURSDAY 8/25/2011	Average (9): 165mg/dL	Carbs: 198g	Insulin: 36.7U Bolus: 58%
FRIDAY 8/26/2011	Average (12): 115mg/dL	Carbs: 174g	Insulin: 30.0U Bolus: 48%
SATURDAY 8/27/2011	Average (9): 148mg/dL	Carbs: 279g	Insulin: 36.0U Bolus: 57%

other. A trend graph has your blood glucose values along the vertical axis and the time of day along the horizontal axis. The horizontal axis generally shows 24 hours and can start at either 5:00 A.M. or midnight, depending on which pump, CGM, or meter you use. Customizable target ranges can be set and are shown as a shaded horizontal bar through the whole graph. Multiple days are represented on the graph as different colored lines with small symbols at each blood glucose value. On a CGM graph, the colored lines are more fluid, with no individual symbols because there are many, many more data points. There is usually also a dotted line that runs through the graph as an average of all the days' values.

Trend graphs make it easy to spot repeating patterns. Trend graphs are also helpful because you can see your highest and lowest values on the graph, and with the adjustable target range you can also see how often your values swing outside this range.

The graph generated by CGM shows a spike of numbers beginning around 4:00 A.M. This graph offers a good visualization of the dawn phenomenon (it is circled in the graph on the next page). The dawn phenomenon occurs when certain hormone levels, such as cortisol and growth hormone, spike in the early morning hours, resulting in increased blood glucose levels, which in turn requires a higher insulin dosage. Looking at this graph will help you identify the dawn phenomenon and allow you to treat it by increasing your early morning basal rate.

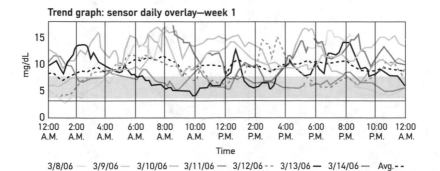

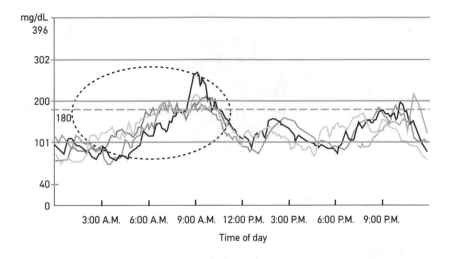

Pie Charts

Pie charts show the averages for the numbers in your target range, above it, and below it. Each pie chart represents a different time of day (e.g., before and after breakfast) or a specific day. Generally, each section is a different color, making it easy to see that a majority of your values are in a certain range. Ideally, you should aim for as much time in the target range as possible, but many people have difficulty achieving more than 50–60% of the time in that range. Similarly, you should aim for as little time in the hypoglycemia range as is possible. Many people have difficulty achieving less than 11% of their values as lows.

Although pie charts identify times when there are too many values in the high or low range, they don't show you the most extreme values. Neither do they show you the standard deviation (covered in this chapter).

Data Tables

These are grids of numbers representing everything, including highest and lowest numbers, standard deviation, averages, number of times glucose testing was performed, frequency of infusion set changes, and percentage above and below target during the days you've selected for review. These types of tables work better with more data points and therefore are good when CGM is used.

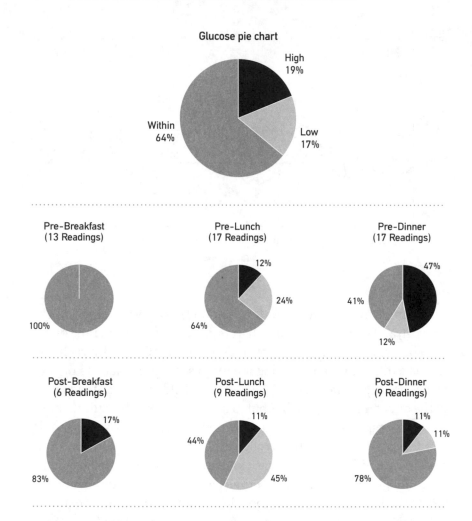

Average Numbers

Average numbers are used to determine glucose levels during specific times of day, such as when you first wake up or when you go to sleep. Averages don't show the highest or lowest numbers (for example, after lunch for the past two weeks).

Standard Deviation

The standard deviation assesses how frequently you go above or below your target range. The standard deviation is the amount, on average, that you swing above or below your target. If your standard deviation number is 35, then that is the average of your high and low numbers and you swing 35 mg/dL above target and 35 mg/dL below target. Optimally, standard deviation numbers should be less than 55 mg/dL or less than half of your average glucose level. For example, if your average glucose is 156, your standard deviation should be less than 78. The purpose of the standard deviation is to give you an idea of the variability within your blood glucose numbers. It is not beneficial to have a high degree of glucose variability.

Percent (%) High, Low, and in Range

The data sheet also shows the percentage (%) of glucose values in the high, low, and target range, just like the pie charts, but these are numerical values rather than graphic representations. These data can be used like the pie charts, and target ranges can be customized for each individual.

At Your Diabetes Appointment

When you see your health care team, team members may download the information from your pump at the clinic, or they may ask you to bring in your own downloaded data. With these tools, they can help you identify areas of optimal and less-than-optimal glucose control and help you determine a course of action. While a lot of focus goes into areas of improvement, it is just as important to celebrate when you have good averages, low standard deviations, and lots of in-range values.

Ultimately, the more you review your data, the better your diabetes control should be. Regularly uploading and reviewing the information stored in your pump will enable you to make changes in your pump settings and diabetes regimen at your health care visits and during the months in between.

PATCH PUMPS AND PUMPS IN THE FUTURE

Patch pumps have no tubing. The actual computer, with its memory, alarms, history, and bolus calculator, is contained within a separate

REMEMBER!

Taking your insulin 15–30 minutes before you eat can be an effective way to improve highs after meals. If you tried to increase your basal rates and/or your ICRs and it caused you to drop to a low value after your initial postprandial (after-meal) spike, then your original dosing values were correct. You may just need to try taking your insulin earlier and have the food "chase" the insulin rather than the other way around.

controller-style device. The controller also contains the blood glucose meter. The "pod" is where the insulin reservoir is filled using a separate needle device. Once the pod is filled, you attach it to your skin with adhesive. Once it is in place, the pod does some automatic checks to make sure everything is working properly and then connects to the controller. After it's connected to the controller, you tell it to insert the cannula. The pod injects the cannula and then retracts the needle automatically. Once the pod is empty, you remove it and throw the whole thing away.

There are many pumps in development with many potential innovations. These innovations might include more-advanced screens, smaller size, more-advanced controllers, and, with continuous glucose monitoring, the ability to automate insulin delivery. This will hopefully lead to the artificial pancreas in the future.

CHAPTER REVIEW

➡ Understanding the components of the pump, the hardware, and the software, as well as the ability to download and interact with glucose monitors and a CGM, is important.

➡ The pump has many functions. It has alarms to notify you. It is critical to understand insulin on board or active insulin, as well as how much the pump bolus calculators can do to help with diabetes management.

➡ The value of looking at your data—at home and during your clinic visits— is immense. Learn the different reports and decide which ones help you the most. Look at patterns and trends and at your behaviors (i.e., your number of boluses and glucose measurements) and keep making improvements.

CHAPTER 4

ALL ABOUT BASAL RATES

WHAT CAN BASAL RATES DO?

One of the great advantages of the insulin pump is that it can be pre-programmed to have one or more basal rates. Basal rates allow for a constant, but variable, amount of insulin to always be present in the blood. This mimics what the pancreas does in people who do not have diabetes; the pancreas always releases some amount of insulin into the bloodstream.

To remind you, basal rates do the job of long-acting insulin in multiple daily injections (MDI)—that's why it's often called basal insulin. In MDI, basal insulins cannot be adjusted during the day, whereas basal rates in the pump can be adjusted or fine-tuned throughout the day and night. This is because pumps use only rapid-acting insulin that is dosed in small, continuous amounts as opposed to long-acting insulin, which is provided only one or two times per day in MDI. If you routinely have physical activity in the afternoon, basal rates can be lowered when insulin requirements are lower. Or if you don't get a lot of physical activity in the morning, then basal rates can be set higher during these hours. Adjustable basal rates also help combat the dawn phenomenon. The dawn phenomenon occurs when certain hormone levels, such as cortisol and growth hormone, spike in the early morning hours, and as a result, blood glucose levels rise and higher amounts of insulin are needed. The advantage of a pump is that it can be programmed to give higher or lower doses of insulin for different parts of the day to more effectively cover activity levels, eating patterns, and other events, like the dawn phenomenon.

Number of Basal Rates

How many different basal rates should you have? This should be determined by you and your health care team. When you first start on an insulin pump, you may have only one or two rates initially programmed into your pump. However, over the first days or weeks of using an insulin pump, your number of basal rates will likely be adjusted to improve your glucose control. Typically, people end up on two to six basal rates per 24-hour time period.

Adjusting and Suspending Basal Rates

The pump's basal rate can be turned off, decreased, or increased for a period of time to compensate for a sudden, perhaps unexpected, change in glucose levels that results from activity, eating, stress, illness, or other factors. For example, if you plan to exercise for an hour at moderate intensity, but actually end up with two hours of high-intensity exercise, then you are at risk for hypoglycemia (because exercise can lower your blood glucose, so the basal insulin rate would send your levels even lower). To protect against hypoglycemia, you could suspend your pump for 30 minutes, decrease the basal insulin delivery by 50% for one hour, or use a combination of both. Conversely, if you need more insulin during a sick day, a long car trip, an extended study session, or your period (many teenage girls and young women need more insulin before, during, or after menstruation), then increasing your basal rate can bring your numbers back into the target range.

Determining exactly how long the pump should be suspended or how much basal rates should be increased or decreased takes some practice. It is helpful to keep a log of how and when you alter your basal rates, so you can understand your own pattern.

GOOD TIMES TO CONSIDER SUSPENDING YOUR PUMP

- During and after exercise
- When you have moderate to severe hypoglycemia, particularly at night
- When your glucose level is rapidly falling, to avoid hypoglycemia

DETERMINING YOUR BASAL RATE NUMBER AND DOSAGE

Determining the appropriate number and dosage of your basal rates is important. It is important when you first start on an insulin pump, and it is important to know that you and your diabetes team will likely keep changing these over time. This is particularly true in children and teenagers as they grow and go through puberty because children have more variation in their eating and physical activity patterns when compared with adults. So don't be surprised that basal rate adjustments are a routine part of insulin pump therapy. After all, you were always adjusting the dosages of insulin you took when you were on injection therapy.

Total Basal Dosage

How much should your total basal dosage be, compared with your total daily dosage (called the total daily insulin dose or TDD)?

The basal rate typically accounts for between 35 and 50% of a person's TDD. Some people need a greater basal rate percentage (perhaps up to 60%) if they eat a very-low-carbohydrate diet, are very sedentary, or have some other issues. However, some people end up with a higher total basal insulin percentage if they do not take enough boluses of insulin every day—perhaps they forget to routinely bolus for meals (lunch is the most commonly forgotten bolus at school) or don't correct enough for high blood glucose levels. This can account for a slow increase in basal rates to respond to insufficient bolusing. So, to understand the basal percentage, it must also be compared with the TDD.

The STAR 3 study (discussed in chapter 1) showed that adults on an insulin pump with a CGM typically split their TDD between the basal and bolus insulin doses almost equally (less than 50% basal, greater than 50% bolus). Children and teens on an insulin pump with a CGM used about 35–40% basal and 60–65% bolus in their TDDs.

Initial Basal Dosage

Your initial basal dosage is determined by averaging the total amount of all the insulins you use each day for about a week. This amount will be a total of your rapid-acting insulin, any intermediate-acting insulin (NPH), and the long-acting or basal insulin. This total is then decreased by about 20–30% because people typically use less insulin when they're on a pump. Then 40–50% of that number becomes the total of all basal rates (some teams start with even less for the total basal rates). Divide that number, the total of all basal rates, by 24 (for the hours in a day) and you have an hourly rate. Of course, this hourly rate can still be adjusted further depending on any particular patterns or issues.

Another way to calculate the basal dosage is by using body weight. Take your weight in kilograms (your weight in pounds divided by 2.2) and multiply that by 0.7. A 135-pound person would weigh 61.3 kilograms. Multiplying your weight in kilograms by 0.7 will give you the TDD. In this instance, that's about 43 units of insulin a day. After calculating this, determining the hourly rate follows the same process.

Through the process of evaluating and fine-tuning you will learn when you need more or less basal insulin. You and your diabetes health care team might decide to have two basal rates at the beginning. You might decide to increase the basal rate in the time between 3:00 and 6:00 A.M. to compensate for the dawn phenomenon. Conversely, you may decide to decrease your basal rate in the afternoon, from 3:00 to 5:00 P.M., when you are physically active. Or you might increase the basal rate in the morning because you usually have high glucose levels between breakfast and lunch.

HOW TO DO BASAL RATE CHECKS

To understand how to adjust basal rates, you can perform basal rate checks. This can be a valuable exercise to do when you first go on the insulin pump. But it can be even more valuable to do basal rate checks after you have been on the pump for a while. In fact, periodic

CALCULATING BASAL RATES: AN EXAMPLE

Lauren is on MDI, taking 15 units of long-acting insulin in the evening and about 20 units of rapid-acting insulin per day. She's starting on an insulin pump. What would her basal rate be?

1. Calculate TDD.

Add up all of her units of insulin per day.

15 + 20 = 35 (TDD)

2. Calculate insulin pump TDD.

Decrease her TDD by 20% because she will probably need less insulin on the pump. Rather than calculating 20% of the TDD and subtracting it, you can simply multiply the TDD by the remaining percentage, which is 80% (100 – 20 = 80%, or 0.80 in decimal).

35 x 0.80 = 28 units

3. Calculate total daily basal dosage.

Lauren will use 40–50% of her TDD for basal insulin. In this example, we'll be conservative and begin with the lowest rate, which is 40%. Multiply her insulin pump TDD by 0.40.

28 x 0.40 = 11.2

Round this down to 11 units of total basal dosage.

4. Calculate the hourly basal rate.

You know how much basal insulin Lauren will need for the day, so we just need to divide that amount by the number of hours in the day to know her hourly rate.

11 ÷ 24 = 0.458

Round this to 0.45 per hour.

Lauren will begin her basal rate at 0.45 unit of insulin per hour.

YOUR INSULIN PUMP SETTINGS

Basal Rates

1. _____ to _____ at units/hour

2. _____ to _____ at units/hour

3. _____ to _____ at units/hour

Bolus Dosages

1. ICRs

1 unit for _____ grams of carbohydrate from _____ to _____ (time)

1 unit for _____ grams of carbohydrate from _____ to _____ (time)

2. Correction Dosages

ISF

1 unit for every ____ mg/dL out of the target range from_____ to _____ (time)

1 unit for every ____ mg/dL out of the target range from_____ to _____ (time)

basal rate checks will help you continue to fine-tune your pump settings and maximize your glucose control.

You check your basal rates by avoiding carbohydrate intake during a set period, so you do not have to give a food bolus. Basal rate checks are done when your blood glucose is between 80 and 140 mg/dL or 90 and 150 mg/dL (i.e., your target range, so you don't have to correct a high or low). To see if there is a pattern, you check each basal rate several times. If there is a dramatic dip in your blood glucose while you are checking the first basal rate, change the basal rate to address the low and check that new basal rate.

The first period to be checked is from 7:00 P.M. to 7:00 A.M. You will need to check and log your glucose level every one to two hours before you go to bed and then every three hours overnight (such as midnight, 3:00 A.M., and 6:00 A.M.). You do this to determine whether you are experiencing overnight lows and highs.

Next, check your morning rates (7:00 A.M. to noon) so you can see what happens to your glucose level if you occasionally sleep in late, delay or miss breakfast, or have a different schedule for weekends and vacations. During this check, skip breakfast and check and record your blood glucose every one or two hours.

You'll check your afternoon rates (noon to 7:00 P.M.) next. Skip lunch and check your blood glucose every one or two hours. If these intervals do not fit your schedule, then you can check for shorter periods or you can divide the overnight, morning, and afternoon periods differently (e.g., 10:00 A.M. to 4:00 P.M. for afternoon).

BEFORE YOU START BASAL RATE CHECKS...

- You want to check your typical blood glucose pattern, so avoid situations that affect your glucose levels, like eating, exercise, stress, menstruation, alcohol consumption, and illness.
- Start four hours after your last bolus, not any earlier.
- The last meal before you do a basal rate check must have a known amount of carbohydrates so that you can accurately dose yourself for the meal. Prepackaged meals are a good choice.
- Don't do an evaluation if you had a severe low blood glucose earlier in the day.

DURING YOUR BASAL RATE CHECKS...

- Frequent blood glucose checks (every one to two hours) are the most important part of these tests! Make sure you check frequently and log all of your results, so that your diabetes care provider can help you determine any rate changes. Or use a CGM.
- If your blood glucose increases or decreases by more than 30–40 mg/dL during the check, STOP the check and treat the glucose level. If this happens, record it and make sure to tell your doctor.
- Drink water.
- Don't do more than one basal rate check a day.
- Don't stress! This test is to help you fine-tune your care, but if something prevents you from doing a check on the day you originally planned, don't worry. Another day will work too.

WHAT ABOUT A CGM?

Because these evaluations require a large number of glucose values, a CGM can be very helpful. If you use a CGM, basal rate checks can be done much easier than with fingersticks.

Don't expect that your basal rates will be *perfect*. Nothing will work 100% of the time. You are looking for what works *most* of the time. Look for trends and patterns rather than focusing on specific numbers.

At the beginning of pump therapy, it may not seem easy. Investing more time and effort in the beginning will pay off with less work and better glucose control later. The occasional reevaluation will need to be done for things like daily activity level changes, pregnancy, weight loss or gain, and aging (teenagers often need more insulin during puberty), but for the most part, your basal rates will not change much. Everyday life will seem a little bit easier, and you'll feel better because you're in good control.

DIFFERENT TYPES OF BASAL RATES

You can switch between your standard basal pattern and a different preprogrammed basal pattern. Or you can use a temporary basal rate. Basal rates can be temporarily increased or decreased for things like exercise, travel, menstruation, or illness.

Basal Patterns

The basal rates you use for a specific situation are called a basal pattern. The basal pattern that you use most of the time is called your standard pattern. This is the pattern you use most of the time, for your everyday, regular life. But you can preprogram other patterns that you use often, such as sick-day patterns, high patterns, low patterns, weekend patterns, and so on. The names of the patterns in some pumps are listed as "A" and "B," but regardless of name, they are set up to have a similar kind of function. There are a number of ways to think about these alternative basal patterns. Some people have a pattern that is a 20% increase (or 120%) in basal rate over the standard pattern. This is useful for sick days, long travel days with limited activity, or menstruation. Another pattern might be a 20% decrease (80%) of the standard pattern that can be used for days of high activity or consistent low blood glucose. Any of these patterns can be used for any amount of time.

> The most common rationale for having two patterns: one for weekdays and one for weekends or holidays, when you are more (or less) active.

Temporary Basal Rates

The other type of basal rate is a temporary basal rate. Temporary basal rates are used for changing basal rate insulin delivery for a fixed period and when you don't want to use a preprogrammed pattern. The temporary basal rate can be set for 24 hours or less. For example, if you are going to go on a long bike ride, you might decrease your normal basal rate by 30% (making your temporary basal rate 70% of the standard pattern) for three hours. Once the three hours are over, the pump automatically goes to the standard basal rate pattern.

Suspend Basal Insulin Delivery

You can also completely suspend insulin delivery for a period of time. You might consider suspending basal insulin during exercise, when you have moderate or severe hypoglycemia, or when your glucose level is falling rapidly (confirmed by multiple glucose measurements or CGM). The pump will indicate that your insulin delivery has been suspended.

ADJUSTING YOUR BASAL RATES

When you are ready to start adjusting your basal rates, you should work very closely with your health care team. To adjust your basal rates, you need the information from your basal rate checks. Data from your pump will be helpful in understanding recurring glucose patterns.

It is very important that changes in your basal rates are made slowly and in small increments. Making dramatic changes to the basal rate can lead to hypoglycemia. For young children, the change in basal rates should be small, such as 0.025–0.05 unit per hour; for teens and adults, 0.1–0.2 unit per hour will work. Once you make a change, wait three to six days before evaluating the results. If you are still experiencing periods of high or low blood glucose, make another small change. However, if you are having frequent, significant lows, it's best to make changes at a faster rate.

Do not try to change several things at once. If you have high morning values and high values before dinner, pick one to work on. It is usually preferable to work on the overnight and then the morning issues first and then work through the rest of the day in order. This is because changes earlier in the day may affect later time periods. Once that change has been made and you no longer are dealing with that issue, start working slowly on the other area. If you are having lows, address those first.

CHAPTER REVIEW

➡ Basal insulin delivery is a key advantage of insulin pump therapy.

➡ Determining your basal rate dosages is done with formulas. Usually you start with one or two basal rates and adjust from there. Overall, total basal dosage is 50% or less of your total daily insulin dose (TDD).

➡ Learn how to do basal rate checks, and do them. It may seem complicated when you first start, but assessing how your basal rates are working is very important.

➡ There are different types of basal rates, called basal patterns. You have your standard pattern, which you use most often. However, you might want different basal rate patterns for weekends and weekdays, for when you are running high or low, when you travel, or have changes in your routine, such as when you are menstruating. Using temporary basal rates can be very helpful, particularly for exercise, stress, and illness.

➡ You should remember that basal rates might change over time. What works now might not work in the future.

CHAPTER 5

ALL ABOUT BOLUSES

There are two kinds of boluses. A bolus dose of insulin can be delivered to bring a high glucose level back into the target range. This is called a correction bolus. A bolus can also be delivered to "cover" food (mainly carbohydrate). This is called a food or mealtime bolus. Of your TDD, 50–65% is usually delivered as bolus insulin each day.

THE CORRECTION BOLUS

A correction bolus is given when your glucose is above the upper level of the target range. This is the range of glucose levels set by your diabetes team that will keep your diabetes in good control. You want your glucose numbers in the target range as much of the time as possible. For adults, the American Diabetes Association (ADA) recommends a glucose range of 70–130 mg/dL before meals and less than 180 mg/dL after meals for many adults, though these numbers should be individualized by the health care team. The more you can keep your glucose in range, the better your A1C levels will be. (Your A1C gives you a three-month average of your glucose levels.) The amount of insulin in your correction bolus will change depending on how high your blood glucose level is. Figuring out how many units to take to bring your glucose back into the target range is calculated using your ISF.

ISF

Your ISF determines how many milligrams per deciliter (mg/dL) 1 unit of insulin will decrease your glucose level. For example, if 1 unit of insulin is expected to bring your glucose down by 50 mg/dL, your ISF ratio would be written as 1:50. You may already be familiar with your ISF from MDI therapy.

Using Your ISF to Correct Blood Glucose Levels

Use your target range to figure out how many units of insulin it will take to bring your glucose back into your range. First, find a number in the middle of your range to use as a target number for your calculations. If your target range is 80–120 mg/dL, for example, pick a number in the middle of the range and calculate from there. To calculate your correction bolus with a target range of 80–120 mg/dL, you could use a target of 100 mg/dL. For practice, pretend you just tested and your glucose is 200 mg/dL and your ISF is 1:50. You can calculate your units of correction insulin by subtracting your target glucose (in this case, 100 mg/dL) from your current blood glucose (in this case, 200 mg/dL). Then you divide your answer by your ISF in order to figure out how much insulin you need to get back to your target of 100 mg/dL.

The equation for a blood glucose reading of 200 mg/dL and an ISF of 1:50 would look like this:

200 – 100 = 100
100 ÷ 50 = 2
Total correction bolus = 2 units

Calculating Your ISF

You're probably wondering how you find out your ISF in the first place. Your diabetes team will help you calculate your first ISF when you're starting on insulin pump therapy. But you can also calculate it yourself. The process starts with the 1700 Rule or the 2000 Rule. If you need more insulin to bring your glucose down, you will use the 1700 Rule. If you need less insulin to bring your glucose down, then you can use the 2000 Rule.

In this example, we will use the 1700 Rule. Start by dividing 1700 by the TDD you use for your pump. Your TDD is 34 units.

$1700 \div 34 = 50$

This means that you will need approximately 1 unit of insulin to bring your blood glucose down 50 mg/dL, which would make your ISF 1:50 (if you get a number that is not whole, just round to the nearest whole number). As with all starting doses that are based on formulas, you will need to closely monitor your glucose levels and perform specific checks to fine-tune the initial settings.

ISFs are not stagnant; they can change over time. They may need to be adjusted when you get older, change activity levels, go through puberty, etc. The way to know whether your ISF is correct is to be aware of how your body reacts to your correction doses and to notice patterns of highs or lows. Many people notice that they are less sensitive to insulin in the morning (during the dawn phenomenon), so they will need more insulin in the morning than in the afternoon or evening. For example, the morning ratio might be 1:40, compared with 1:50 for the afternoon and evening. It is important to understand that "less sensitive" means 1 unit of insulin will bring you down a lower number of milligrams per deciliter (mg/dL) in the glucose level; thus, it will take more units of insulin to get you into the desired range (for example, the less-sensitive ratio of 1:40 means that to come from 250 to 100 mg/dL, you will need 3.8 units of insulin). "More sensitive" means 1 unit of insulin will bring you down a greater amount in the glucose level (for example, the more-sensitive ratio of 1:50 means that to come from 250 to 100 mg/dL, you will need 3.0 units of insulin).

Some people have two or even three ISFs for a 24-hour period. Insulin pumps will remember your different ratios and use them in you pump bolus calculator at the appropriate times.

Checking and Evaluating Your ISF

As with the evaluation of basal rates, you need to verify that your ISFs are right for you. You accomplish this by checking them. You do ISF checks after you have corrected a high glucose level and when you have the ability to see how the correction bolus brings your glucose level down without other factors affecting it. For example, you can do an ISF check when you have not eaten carbohydrates for three to four hours and don't have any active insulin from a previous food bolus. You also do ISF checks when you have not exercised, been ill, or been stressed for at least three to four hours (or had alcohol for 24 hours).

When you find that it has been three to four hours since your last meal and your glucose is elevated out of the target range, you can do an ISF check. Give your correction bolus, and check your glucose levels every one to two hours after the initial correction bolus. Record your results.

If three to four hours have passed since your correction bolus and you are not back in your target range, you might consider repeating this procedure on another day. If you have the same results on a second test, you might want to consider changing your ISF in the pump settings.

Examples
If your ISF is 1:50 and your glucose is 250 mg/dL, you would take 3 units to bring your glucose to 100 mg/dL (250 − 100 = 150; 150 ÷ 50 = 3). If your glucose was 167 mg/dL at four hours during your ISF check, then you need to change the ratio, because the correction bolus has not sufficiently lowered your blood glucose. You could try 1:40, so you'd need 3.8 units (150 ÷ 40 = 3.75, rounded to 3.8). You change your ISF because you need *more* insulin to lower your blood glucose to the desired level. You could also try an ISF of 1:45, which would mean that you would have taken 3.3 units to correct (150 ÷ 45 = 3.33, rounded to 3.3).

Conversely, if your blood glucose is lower than target at any point during your ISF check, you may need to change your ISF in the opposite direction. In this case, you might want to change from 1:50 to 1:70. Therefore, you would have taken 2.1 units for this correction (150 ÷ 70 = 2.14, rounded to 2.1). This is because you need less insulin to bring your glucose down.

BOLUSES FOR FOOD

Insulin boluses regulate glucose levels in response to the foods and drinks you consume, especially when they contain carbohydrate (sometimes called carbs or written as CHO). Carbohydrates are broken down into sugar molecules, which are used as fuel by your cells. Insulin allows this sugar to enter into the cells. Because a person with diabetes does not have enough insulin in his or her body or because the body is more resistant to the effects of insulin, insulin injections must be used to replace insulin. These mealtime doses of insulin are called boluses, and a bolus is given as an injection or by the push of buttons on an insulin pump.

ICR

The bolus calculator in the insulin pump can calculate the amount of insulin needed for the amount of carbohydrate ingested. First, you have to determine what your ICR is, if you don't already have one.

Calculating Your ICR

To determine your ICR, most people use the 450 Rule. The 450 Rule is similar to the 1700 or the 2000 Rule for determining ISF. You divide 450 by your insulin TDD. Let's use the same example we used for calculating ISF, when the TDD was 34. If your TDD is 34, then $450 \div 34 = 14.7$ (you can round to the nearest whole number if needed, in this case to 15), so 1 unit of insulin is needed for every 15 grams of carbohydrate ingested. The ICR equals 1:15.

Some people might have several ICRs throughout the day. Some people have a different ICR at breakfast than for the rest of the day. This is because insulin sensitivity may be decreased in the morning, so more insulin is required per gram of carbohydrate than for meals later in the day. For example, an ICR at breakfast may be 1:12, whereas it may be 1:15 during the rest of the day.

You might already have had an ICR from when you were on MDI therapy. These ICRs might change in response to being on insulin pump therapy. It is a good idea to recalculate and reevaluate your ICRs.

Checking and Evaluating Your ICR
You can check whether your ICR is correct, just like you can check your basal rates and your ISF. You accomplish this by doing ICR checks. You can check your ICR when you have a glucose reading before eating that is in the target range and when you can accurately calculate the amount of carbohydrate you are ingesting (in food and beverages). This gives you the ability to see how the ICR works for your food and beverages without other factors affecting it. For example, make sure to do ICR checks when you have not had to correct a high glucose value for three to four hours and when you don't have bolus insulin that is still active from previous food boluses or correction doses. Also, do ICR checks when you have not exercised, been ill, or been stressed for at least three to four hours (or had alcohol for 24 hours), just like when you check your ISF.

After the food bolus (determined by the bolus calculator) is given, check your glucose every hour for four hours. The ADA recommends that post-meal blood glucose levels be below 180 mg/dL in adults at 2–3 hours. If, during the four hours after eating (without more food or exercise), your glucose reading is back in the target range, then the ICR is correct. If, after three to four hours, your blood glucose is above the target range, then the ICR should be changed to give more insulin per gram of carbohydrate. If your glucose is below the target, then your ICR should be changed to give less insulin per gram of carbohydrate. There is one other issue: if at four hours your blood glucose is in the target range, but there were values higher than 180 mg/dL in between, you might need to think about the timing of your insulin bolus for food. Taking your insulin 15–30 minutes before you begin eating improves your control.

Here are two examples. If your ICR is 1:15 and you ingest 60 grams of carbohydrate for lunch, then you'll take 4 units of insulin to cover the meal (60 ÷ 15 = 4). If at four hours your glucose is 225 mg/dL, then you need to *decrease* your ICR. You can try a new ICR of 1:12. You would then take 5 units of insulin for a 60-gram carbohydrate meal (60 ÷ 12 = 5). This is because you need *more* insulin to keep your glucose level in the target range after eating. If you tried a new ICR of 1:10, then you would take 6 units of insulin (60 ÷ 10 = 6).

Conversely, if your glucose is lower than target at any point within four hours after your meal, you may need to *increase* your ICR. You might want to change from 1:15 to 1:18, for example. In that case, you would have taken 3.3 units (60 ÷ 18 = 3.33). This is because you need less insulin to cover your meal.

Timing the Food Bolus

In general, it is best to give the insulin bolus 15–30 minutes before eating. It takes about 15 minutes for carbohydrate to start to influence your blood glucose levels, with peak effects around 60 minutes after eating. Even rapid-acting insulin takes longer to start working, reaching its peak effect at 90–100 minutes after a bolus.

With young children, it is often difficult to determine how much they will eat. It has been shown that giving insulin after the meal can still allow for good diabetes control. If you do this, and the young child decides to eat less, you will not have given them too much insulin. However, for the most part, it is better to give a little insulin before eating and then play "catch up" as food is consumed. For example, if a young child usually eats 22 grams of carbohydrate for breakfast and has an ICR of 1:20, then you can guess that the child will probably need 1.1 units of insulin (22 ÷ 20 = 1.1). You can give a fraction of this dose before the meal, such as 0.2–0.4 unit, and then give the rest as the child is eating or when the meal is completed. This is a major advantage of an insulin pump, because it is easy to give some insulin before the meal if you are not comfortable giving the full dose in advance.

Bolusing for Carbohydrates and Correction

When you are ready to eat a meal or snack or drink something with carbohydrate, you should check your glucose before you start eating or drinking and count the carbohydrates you're going to consume. Your glucose before you eat or drink will be within your target range, above your target range, or below your target range.

Within Target Range
If your glucose is in the target range, then you take insulin to cover the carbohydrate.

Above Target Range
If your glucose is higher than your target, you have two choices. You can correct the elevated glucose first and wait 30 minutes or more until your glucose comes back into the target range. Or you can take a bolus that adds the correction dose of insulin to the dose you are going to take to cover your carbohydrates. If you do this, you should wait 15–30 minutes after the bolus before you start eating in order to allow your glucose level to start to come down first.

Below Target Range
If your glucose level is below target before you start to eat—in the hypoglycemic range—what should you do? There are a few options.

- Consume 15 grams of carbohydrate to correct your glucose level before you eat (if your child is younger than 10 years of age, you might want to give only 8 grams) and wait 15 minutes. Check your blood glucose. If it is still low, consume another 15 grams of carbohydrate and check again 15 minutes later. Repeat this process until you are back in the target range. This is called the Rule of 15. Once your blood glucose is back in the target range, you can take your insulin dose to cover the carbohydrate in your meal. This is particularly helpful if you were going to eat a high-fat meal, because a lot of fat will slow the effects of carbohydrate on your blood glucose levels.

- Decrease your insulin bolus using the pump's bolus calculator. For example, if your target range is 90–100 mg/dL and your glucose is 70 mg/dL before you plan to eat a 45-gram carbohydrate meal, you can use the bolus calculator's settings to estimate a dose that subtracts some insulin, taking into account that your blood glucose is a little low.

- Decrease your insulin bolus by considering some of the carbohydrate you are about to eat as "free" (meaning that it will not be treated with insulin). So if your ICR is 1:15, you would normally take 3 units of insulin for a 45-gram carbohydrate meal. For example, if your pre-meal glucose is 60 mg/dL, it is recommended that you ingest 15 grams of carbohydrate as "free." So you subtract 15 from 45, and use only 30 grams of the carbohydrate that you are going to eat in calculating your meal bolus. This means you would only take 2 units of insulin for the meal. You might even consider waiting until after you have started eating and the food has begun to elevate your glucose level before taking the full bolus.

Bolus Types

There are different types of food boluses. These different boluses can extend the time over which the bolus is delivered by your pump.

Regular Bolus

A regular bolus delivers all of the insulin over a short period of time. The amount of time it takes depends on how fast the pump motor can give the dose.

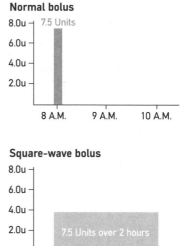

Normal bolus

7.5 Units

8.0u
6.0u
4.0u
2.0u

8 A.M.   9 A.M.   10 A.M.

Square-Wave or Extended Bolus

A square-wave (or extended) bolus dispenses insulin over a specified amount of time. This is good for high-fat meals because the stomach empties more slowly after a high-fat meal, and a regular bolus of insulin might cause blood glucose levels to go low. This bolus can also be used for long periods of snacking (such as at parties, sporting events, and movies).

Square-wave bolus

8.0u
6.0u
4.0u
2.0u

7.5 Units over 2 hours

8 A.M.   9 A.M.   10 A.M.

Dual-Wave or Combination-Wave Bolus

A dual-wave bolus is a combination of a regular meal bolus, which is given all at once, and the square-wave bolus. This combination is good for high-carb/high-fat meals, like pizza and Chinese or Italian food.

Dual-wave bolus

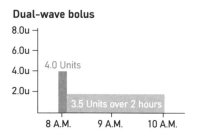

Generally the total calculated bolus is given as 50% in a regular food bolus and 50% in the square-wave bolus. For example, if a 7.5-unit bolus is calculated for a meal, then 4 units will be given at the beginning and 3.5 units will be spread out over a certain amount of time (normally two hours). These figures will vary depending on the individual. Different types of meals might also require different distributions of the bolus (for example, pizza versus Chinese food). Over time, you will figure out which combination works best for you.

THE BOLUS CALCULATOR

Pumps have bolus calculators that make it easier and safer to give more accurate doses. The bolus calculator uses personalized settings that are prescribed by your diabetes team, keeps track of your previous boluses, and does the complicated math to provide an estimated dose. The bolus calculator will provide a suggested dose. It is your responsibility to take into consideration other important factors that could be affecting your insulin requirements (such as exercise or illness) and to decide whether you are going to deliver the suggested dose or adjust the estimate before delivering the dose.

TAKE ADVANTAGE!

Take advantage of your pump's ability to do square-wave or dual-wave boluses. It can be extremely helpful to use these functions. The only way to really know which bolus type will work best for your body and the food you eat is to try these boluses and monitor your blood glucose two and four hours after your meal. Many people will start with a two- or three-hour period of extended delivery. In the case of the dual-wave, take half the needed insulin as a regular bolus and half over an extended period of time. People who use these different bolus methods might find that their blood glucose levels are better managed.

BOLUS CALCULATOR SETTINGS AND INFORMATION

Bolus calculator settings that are programmed into the pump during setup (these may vary at different times of the day and night):

- Blood glucose target range
- ICR
- ISF
- Active insulin time

➡ Your current glucose level is either entered by you or transmitted automatically from your glucose meter.

➡ You enter the number of grams of carbohydrate that you plan to eat each time you give a bolus for food.

ACTIVE INSULIN AND INSULIN ON BOARD

When you are calculating a correction bolus for a high glucose value, you may still have bolus insulin in your system from a previous food or correction bolus. The amount of insulin left in your bloodstream is referred to as active insulin or insulin on board. The amount of active insulin decreases as time passes because your body absorbs the insulin in the bloodstream. Your insulin pump can calculate the remaining active insulin using the active insulin/insulin-on-board setting. It is important to consider the presence of active insulin, because taking a correction bolus on top of active insulin (known as "stacking insulin") can lead to hypoglycemia.

For example, if you ate a big meal and took a bolus 15 minutes before eating, you may still have an elevated glucose level two hours later. If you want to correct this after-meal high, you should not take a full correction dose. You should account for the active insulin that is still in your blood from your meal bolus. If you plan on eating more carbohydrate, you might want to only dispense a bolus for the extra carbs you are going to eat and not add any correction at all. Or you can add a correction dose that is modified by the active insulin. If you choose to give a full correction bolus and a food bolus when you have active insulin in your system two hours after your previous bolus, then you would be stacking insulin and increasing the chances that you'll go low.

The concept of active insulin/insulin on board also applies to correction boluses. If you corrected at noon but your glucose level was higher one hour later, then you would not want to take a full correction bolus for this new higher glucose level because you still have active insulin. Instead, you would take a decreased bolus that accounts for how much active insulin is still in your blood from the first correction bolus.

The pump bolus calculator will calculate all of these different factors together when you enter your blood glucose and the number of carbohydrates you plan to eat. The pump stores all of your ratios for use in these calculations and will also incorporate active insulin. The calculator will suggest a dose, but you are always able to make changes to it (in the event of increased activity, for example).

However, always be sure to check for ketones in situations in which the risk of DKA is present. Pump calculators do not calculate the extra insulin that is needed when someone has ketones (see chapter 9).

CHAPTER REVIEW

➡ Bolusing the right amount at the right time and for the right reasons is a key to success. Correction boluses help manage diabetes and are dependent on obtaining the right ISF. You calculate your ISF with specific formulas, and these may vary throughout the day. Do correction bolus checks to be sure you have the right ISF to bring you back to the target range after a high glucose level and without increasing hypoglycemia.

➡ Food boluses are calculated with formulas, and these may change throughout the day and night. Many people need more insulin for carbohydrate in the morning. You should check and evaluate your ICR to be sure you have the right ratio to manage your diabetes. You need to understand the importance of the timing of food boluses, correctly counting carbohydrate, and determining which bolus—normal, square-wave, or dual-wave—to use.

➡ The bolus calculator provides the huge advantage to insulin pump therapy. The bolus calculator helps determine how much insulin is needed for food and correction boluses.

➡ The bolus calculator also considers active insulin, or insulin on board, to ensure that safe boluses are always delivered. This helps prevent insulin stacking and the resulting hypoglycemia.

IN THIS CHAPTER

- Fixed Meal Plans
- All about Carbs
- The Food Label
- The Importance of Accurate Measurements
- Glycemic Index

CHAPTER 6

UNDERSTANDING THE MEAL PLAN

A healthy, balanced nutrition plan is the key to strong diabetes management. It is important to understand how the foods and beverages you eat and drink affect your glucose levels. It is just as important to understand how much insulin you need to take for what you eat and drink. Carbohydrate is the main nutrient that affects your glucose levels, so you need to learn how to count carbohydrate. But you must also understand how the other macronutrients—fat and protein—interact with carbohydrate, in order to customize your insulin use to your body's individual needs. These are critical skills to have in your journey with diabetes.

FIXED MEAL PLANS

Before the discovery of insulin, the only thing that could be done to help someone with type 1 diabetes survive was to restrict his or her intake of carbohydrates and calories. After the discovery of insulin, people were put on a fixed dietary plan. They were not allowed to have simple carbohydrates (sugars). They were told they needed to eat the same thing—mainly protein, complex carbohydrates, and fat—at the same time every day so that glucose peaks from food could be matched by insulin peaks from one, two, or three injections a day. As a result, people were forced to eat at set times whether they were hungry or not and were not allowed to eat at other times, even if they were hungry. If they ate more or ate during these forbidden times, they were accused of "cheating." The diet was dreary, and following it was not fun for most people with diabetes.

The Exchange Diet

The original fixed diet plan evolved over time into a number of different nutrition plans. One of the most popular plans was called the Exchange diet. The Exchange diet was based on breaking down the components of the diet into "exchanges." In this way you could exchange one food for another provided they both contained a similar amount of nutrients and calories, thereby allowing the diet to be more varied. For example, a carbohydrate could be exchanged for a different carbohydrate of equal quantity, one protein could be exchanged for another protein, and fat could be exchanged for fat. Because carbohydrate management is essential in diabetes, the exchange system focused on carbohydrates. Various carbohydrates were compared to a slice of bread (or 15 grams of carbohydrate), and this was known as one carbohydrate exchange or one "carb choice." An apple, half a banana, a half cup of pasta, and half a baked potato were all one carbohydrate exchange. With the Exchange system, the number of exchanges (or choices) that you were allotted per meal was dictated by your dietitian or health care provider. The Exchange system is no longer the preferred nutrition plan for someone with type 1 diabetes (carb counting is), but its principles are used in weight-management programs because this method highlights nutritional composition and serving size.

In 1995, a few years after the DCCT results were reported and the importance of intensive diabetes management was realized, the Exchange system underwent revision and improvement. It began to be based more on counting carbohydrates. You were no longer obligated to eat carbohydrate in 15-gram portions or in amounts equivalent to an exchange. You could actually start to count individual grams of carbohydrate and link grams of carbohydrate with units of insulin, via the ICR. Once rapid-acting insulin came onto the scene, the world was ready to switch directly to carb counting. And nothing is more suited for carb counting than the insulin pump.

ALL ABOUT CARBS

Carbohydrates are sources of energy—fuel for our bodies. Your gastrointestinal tract breaks down carbohydrate into individual sugar molecules. This group includes starches (bread, pasta, potatoes, cake, etc.) and simple sugars (glucose, lactose, sucrose, and fructose). Carbohydrate even includes fiber.

Types of Carbohydrate

There are three types of carbohydrate, and all affect your blood glucose levels. Starches (complex carbohydrate), sugars (simple carbohydrate), and fiber are all forms of carbohydrate. Starch and sugar cause blood glucose levels to spike and generally have a higher glycemic index (covered later in this chapter). Foods high in complex carbohydrate (i.e., starches) include vegetables, such as potatoes, corn, and winter squash, but also include grains, pasta, breads, cereals, cookies, cakes, and more. Simple sugar acts quickly and is found in foods like honey, milk, syrup, table sugar, fruit, and fruit juices.

Each gram of starch or sugar counts as a gram of carbohydrate. So if you eat a small apple, it has 15 grams of carbohydrate. A piece of bread has 15 grams, as does one serving of pasta (½ cup). A serving of cereal might be 15 or 22 grams, depending on the size.

Fiber, even though it is a carbohydrate, is a bit different. Your body can't break down all fiber. Therefore, fiber is never fully converted to glucose. If a large portion of the total carbohydrate in your meal comes from fiber (generally about 5 or more grams of fiber) you can reduce the number of carbs you're counting in your meal by the amount of fiber. For example, if you eat 36 grams of carbs and 7 grams of that is fiber, then you would use 29 grams of carbs to calculate your meal bolus (36 − 7 = 29).

There is evidence that when you are on an insulin pump, it is best to manage your diabetes by using carbohydrate counting (usually shortened to "carb counting" or "counting carbs"). By counting carbs, you know how much insulin to dose. This process is made easier by the fact that food labels are required by law to show you how much carbohydrate is in each serving of food. Reading the food label (which is covered later in this chapter) is important and makes diabetes management easier. With the help of the food label, you can determine the amount of carbohydrate per serving size of the food. When used with your ICR, you can very successfully determine how much insulin is needed to cover a meal. Carb counting, your ICR, and your pump combine to be a very powerful toolbox for managing your diabetes.

Carb Counting

The more accurate you are with your carb counting, the better your diabetes management will be when you use insulin pump therapy. Thankfully, once you know how to read a food label, understand how to measure your portions (with scales, measuring cups, serving spoons, etc.), and can calculate your ICR, determining how much insulin to dose can be a rather straightforward practice. You will need to work with your diabetes team, especially a registered dietitian, to become skilled at carb counting. You will need to learn about basic nutrition and read some carb-counting books so you can make healthy choices at your meals and snacks.

At first, this may be somewhat daunting—calculating and precisely measuring every food you eat never sounds like a lot of fun. But like so many other things about starting on a pump, it will become routine and you will eventually remember the carb content of the foods you eat most often, as well as what constitutes a serving size. The benefits of your diligence in the beginning will definitely pay off in the long run.

FOR YOUR REFERENCE

An excellent guide to the skills of carb counting is the *Complete Guide to Carb Counting*, 3rd edition, by Hope S. Warshaw and Karmeen Kulkarni, published by the American Diabetes Association.

THE FOOD LABEL

Reading a food label is a key skill for managing blood glucose levels and carb counting successfully. Start reading them now. There are four things that you must always look at when you read a nutrition or food label. These are

- serving size

- total fat

- total carbohydrates

- dietary fiber

Let's look at a food label together. The example we will use is for a blueberry bagel. The best idea is to start at the top of the food label.

Nutrition Facts
Serving Size 1 bagel (95g)
Servings Per Container 6

Amount Per Serving

Calories 270   Calories from Fat 20

% Daily Value*

Total Fat 2g	3%
Saturated Fat 0.5g	3%
Trans Fat 0g	
Cholesterol 0mg	0%
Sodium 440mg	18%
Total Carbohydrate 54g	18%
Dietary Fiber 3g	12%
Sugars 11g	
Protein 9g	

Vitamin A	0%	•	Vitamin C	0%
Calcium	10%	•	Iron	15%
Thiamin	25%	•	Riboflavin	15%
Niacin	15%	•	Folic Acid	25%

*Percent Daily Values are based on a 2,000 calorie diet. Your Daily Values may be higher or lower depending on your calorie needs.

		Calories:	2,000	2,500
Total Fat	Less than		65g	80g
Sat Fat	Less than		20g	25g
Cholesterol	Less than		300mg	300mg
Sodium	Less than		2,400mg	2,400mg
Potassium			3,500mg	3,500mg
Total Carbohydrate			300g	375g
Dietary Fiber			25g	30g

Calories per gram:
Fat 9   •   Carbohydrate 4   •   Protein 4

Serving Size

What is the serving size here? This label shows the serving size for a whole bagel, but be careful, because sometimes the serving size is just half a bagel. Knowing this is essential because all of the rest of the nutrient content is based on a single serving of the food. The next time you grab a bag of chips, look closely at how many servings are in the bag. The label will tell you right under the serving size. There are six bagels in this bag. Each bagel is one serving. Serving sizes often give the amount in weight as well as volume. Some labels will indicate a measurement, such as ½ cup, as well as a weight in ounces (oz) or grams. In this case, the weight of the entire bagel is 95 grams. These weight grams are different from the grams of carbohydrate in the serving, so be careful not to mix them up! If this label indicated that the serving size is a half bagel, then you'd have to double all of the nutrients in the food label if you eat the whole bagel.

Total Fat

The next thing to look at is total fat. This entire bagel has 2 grams (or 2 g) of fat. If you look at the line right above the total fat line you will see the total calories. Look to the right of total calories, and you will see how many of the calories come from fat. In this case, total calories for one serving are 270, with 20 calories from fat. Overall, you should look for foods in which fat contributes 30% of the total calories or less. In the case of this bagel, that would be more than 80 calories, so 20 calories is really good! You should generally try to eat lower amounts of fat and make sure that saturated fat contributes only about 7% of your total calories per day.

Total Carbohydrate

Total carbohydrate gives you the total amount of carbohydrate, including sugar and fiber, in the food. For this bagel, total carbohydrate is 54 grams. If you were using an ICR of 1:15 (1 unit for every 15 grams of carbohydrate), the total amount of insulin needed to cover this bagel would be 3.6 units (54 ÷ 15= 3.6). If you were still on MDI, you wouldn't be able to take 3.6 units of insulin. You would have to round down to 3.5 units or up to 4 units. With an insulin pump, you can administer these small increments, as low as 0.025 unit. For some people, these small increments are necessary to fine-tune insulin delivery.

When looking at the total carbohydrate content, keep in mind the serving size! If you eat only half the bagel, then you will need to take only half the amount of insulin—1.8 units instead of 3.6 units.

ANOTHER THING ABOUT FAT

Fat delays the emptying of your stomach. So it takes longer for food to digest and have an effect on your glucose level. You might want to consider using a dual-wave or square-wave bolus if you eat high-fat foods (foods with 30% or more calories from fat).

Dietary Fiber

The last thing to look at is the dietary fiber content. This bagel has 3 grams of fiber. It is important to have fiber in your diet, and foods high in fiber are usually healthy choices. Fruits and vegetables are naturally high in fiber. Whole grains contain higher amounts of fiber than processed grains. Because fiber is not digested completely in your gastro-intestinal tract, fiber has little effect on your glucose levels. If you eat a food with more than 5 grams of fiber, you can subtract the grams of fiber from the total grams of carbohydrate for the carb number you will use with your ICR. For example, if the bagel had 7 grams of fiber, you would subtract 7 from 54 to get 47, and 47 would be the total number of carbs you would use in the ICR, which means that you would take 3.1 units of insulin for a bagel with 7 grams of fiber. In general, high-fiber foods don't elevate your blood glucose as much as foods without fiber.

Protein

You should also check the amount of protein in the food you are choosing. Protein is an essential nutrient, but many people eat too much of it. Try to get 20% of your daily calories from protein. If you have kidney disease, you should aim for the lower end of that range.

IF YOU CAN'T FIND A FOOD LABEL

Although the food label is a useful thing to have so that you can more effectively manage your diabetes, not everything has one. When was the last time you saw a food label on fresh fruit, a hamburger, or a restaurant meal? There are many foods that you will encounter every day that will not have a label, but there are other ways to get the nutrition facts you need to help determine your insulin requirements. Most chain and fast-food restaurants have their nutrition facts online and in pamphlets at the restaurant. If you are lucky, those details will be right there on the menu. Sometimes this information is hidden away, but if you ask for it, you can see it. There are many books that have the nutrition facts for a variety of restaurants. Such books are generally small or pocket-size and portable. Bring them with you when you are out and about.

A VALUABLE RESOURCE

In addition to the nearly countless online resources for nutrition information, you can also carry this information with you at all times. Pick up a copy of *The Diabetes Carbohydrate & Fat Gram Guide,* 4th edition, by Lea Ann Holzmeister, published by the American Diabetes Association and the Academy of Nutrition and Dietetics, or *The American Diabetes Association Guide to Healthy Restaurant Eating,* 4th edition, by Hope S. Warshaw, also published by the American Diabetes Association.

Note that there is not enough scientific evidence to suggest that a high-protein, low-carbohydrate diet is helpful in managing diabetes.

THE IMPORTANCE OF ACCURATE MEASUREMENTS

In addition to knowing the number of carbohydrates in each serving of the foods you eat, taking accurate measurements of how much you actually eat is an important part of counting carbs. If the amount you actually eat does not equal what you thought you ate, then your bolus will be incorrect. Measuring is important, but it can definitely be difficult. Here are some tips that will help you get started with measuring accurately:

• Some items need to be measured by weight or by volume. A food scale will be best for weighing things like bread, which generally has 15 grams of carbohydrate in each ounce. A scale can also be used for fruits and pasta—the serving size for pasta is almost always 2 ounces, but it can vary. Measuring cups can be good for grains and cereals, graduated cups are good for liquids (bend down, so that you are eye level with the measurements), and teaspoons and tablespoons are good for jams, honey, butter, and peanut butter.

- Always level off what's in your measuring utensil with a knife.

- Check to see if the food label or the book indicates raw versus cooked, because this distinction can change the composition of the food's nutrition content.

- Watch your portion sizes as you grow more confident in your ability to estimate. If your glucose numbers are rising, go back to carefully measuring your foods. Often, as time passes, we lose track of what a true serving looks like. If this happens to you, it's time to go back and recalibrate your visual measuring skills.

- Start to notice what different foods look like on your plate. This will be helpful when you go out to eat and don't have a measuring cup or scale handy. There are some good ways to estimate size, but it is still important to keep measuring every so often to keep your estimates accurate.

- There are some easy ways to estimate what you're eating by comparing them to objects with which you are very familiar. Using this system, 3 oz of meat is about the size of a deck of playing cards. A ½ cup of pasta, rice, or grains is about the size of your palm, whereas 1 cup is the size of your fist. A medium potato is the size of a computer mouse. With fruits, a "small" piece would be about the size of a tennis ball and ½ cup is about the size of a baseball. A tablespoon of peanut butter and other similar foods is about equal to the size of your thumb. A teaspoon is about the size of the tip of your thumb. A small cup of coffee is about 8 oz or 1 cup of liquid. One ounce of cheese is about the size of three dice.

GLYCEMIC INDEX

The glycemic index is a meal-planning tool based on how quickly the carbohydrates in a food will affect blood glucose levels. Foods are listed on a scale of 1–100, with 100 being a food that affects your blood glucose the fastest. Pure glucose is the fastest carbohydrate in terms of reaching the blood and has a glycemic index of 100. All other foods are compared to this. Low glycemic foods are generally considered 55 and under, whereas high glycemic foods are above 75. Be aware, however, that the glycemic index of a food does not affect the total amount of insulin you take. It is not a carbohydrate count. A slice of sourdough bread has a glycemic index of 52. So do four slices of sourdough bread, but the four slices of bread contain more carbohydrate and will need more insulin to be covered.

Timing of Insulin Delivery

The glycemic index helps you plan the timing of insulin delivery. If you are aware that you will be eating something with a high glycemic index later in the day (say, french fries, which have a count of 75), then taking your insulin 30 minutes before eating it will greatly reduce the risk of a quick spike in blood glucose. It is already a good idea to take your insulin 15–30 minutes before you eat a meal, but taking your insulin early for a meal that is going to have a high glycemic index is particularly effective for managing blood glucose levels. However, foods with a low glycemic index take longer to reach your bloodstream and might need insulin administered over a longer period of time. A square-wave bolus would be a good option here. Pasta, although high in carbohydrates, is low on the glycemic scale, with a count of 41. Foods like pasta (high in carbohydrate and low in glycemic index) are often treated with a dual-wave bolus because an initial burst of insulin is needed to cover the first glucose spike as the food is first digested. But because the carbs will take longer to reach the bloodstream, insulin delivery also will have to be drawn out, making the dual-wave bolus the ideal solution.

Things that affect the glycemic index include fat; any coating on the food, such as waxy beans and legumes; ripeness (the sugar content in many fruits and vegetables increases with age); type of starch; fiber content; acidity (it slows digestion); processing; cooking methods; and your before-meal glucose level. Processed grains have had the bran and germ removed, which reduces the content of natural nutrients like fiber, resulting in a higher glycemic index count. With cooking, the longer you cook a food, the faster it reaches the bloodstream. This is because the cooking process starts to break down the carbohydrate in the food, making it easier for the body to absorb it. So, potatoes already have a very high glycemic index, but if you bake them for a long time, the glycemic index will rise to an even higher number (a baked red-skin potato can be as high as 93).

CHAPTER REVIEW

➡ Carbohydrate counting is the preferred meal-planning tool for someone using an insulin pump. Compared with other methods, counting carbs is easier and more precise, once you determine your ICR.

➡ Carbohydrates come in three forms: starches, sugars, and fiber. A gram of starch or sugar is counted as a gram of carbohydrate. Fiber is counted differently. Fiber is not completely digested or converted to glucose. If there is a large portion of fiber in your meal (five or more grams), then you can subtract the number of grams of fiber from the total carbohydrate count.

➡ There are four key elements to look at when you read a food label. These are serving size, total fat, total carbohydrates, and dietary fiber.

➡ If you do not know how much you eat or drink, you will not be able to accurately calculate how much insulin you need to take. Measuring is important! But measuring is also not always easy because there is not one way that works to measure every food you eat. With practice, you will become familiar with portion sizes.

➡ The glycemic index is based on how quickly the carbohydrates in a food will affect blood glucose levels. Foods are listed on a scale of 1–100, with 100 being the fastest, which is pure glucose. The glycemic index helps you plan the timing of insulin delivery. It is a good idea to take your insulin 15–30 minutes before you eat, but taking insulin early with a high glycemic index meal will help control glucose levels. Foods with a low glycemic index take longer to reach your bloodstream and need insulin to be given over a longer period of time; in cases such as this, a square-wave or dual-wave bolus might be ideal.

CHAPTER 7

UNDERSTANDING THE IMPACT OF PHYSICAL ACTIVITY

Hopefully, you are physically active and have regular exercise as a part of your daily routine. Exercise not only helps your metabolism, but also helps you maintain a healthy weight and is good for your heart, your muscles, your bones, and your mood, whether or not you have diabetes. It doesn't matter if you are an athlete or someone who rarely gets off the couch; managing your diabetes with an insulin pump can make it easier to keep your glucose levels under control with exercise—particularly if your activity varies in intensity and duration from one day to the next. Understanding how to manage planned and unplanned physical activity is important for a successful journey with diabetes and with insulin pump therapy.

To be active doesn't mean you have to run marathons or put in long hours at the gym. You can take a walk at lunch or after school. You can dance, bike to the store, work in your garden, wash your car, and routinely take the stairs instead of the elevator. Even standing for parts of the day instead of sitting will help. Do your best to move your body as much as possible and you and your diabetes will reap the benefits.

GET MOVIN'!

Just 30 minutes of moderate exercise a day at least five times a week is recommended for all people—young or old and everyone in between. With diabetes or without! So get out and get movin' for your health!

JUST STARTING OUT

When you first get your pump and you're trying to determine how to set your bolus and basal rates, you actually don't want to exercise, even if you are someone who exercises routinely. It is easier to determine your pump settings when you are sedentary (i.e., not very physically active). Once you establish your ratios and feel comfortable with your pump, you can start being active again.

Start slowly and exercise for a shorter period of time than usual. For example, if you routinely exercise for 45–60 minutes several times a week, start out at 20–30 minutes. Once you figure out how to manage these shorter periods of activity, you can increase your exercise by 15–20 minutes, until you get to your typical exercise duration. You can do the same with intensity. Start with a lower intensity until you get the hang of how to manage your glucose and insulin levels during exercise. After that, you can move up the intensity ladder. In the end, you will succeed in being active and having optimal glucose control.

Exercise Physiology

Hypoglycemia is a risk of exercise. The more you exercise, the more sensitive to insulin you will become. Being more sensitive to insulin means you might need to take less insulin overall. Exercise helps increase the number of insulin receptors on cells. When insulin attaches to these receptors, glucose can pass from the blood into the cell. This reduces the amount of glucose in the blood, which can lead to hypoglycemia.

Your muscles use carbohydrate and fat. Once food is absorbed and the resulting glucose is used up, your body has to rely on its own stores. At the beginning of exercise, the muscles use their own glucose stores (glucose is stored as glycogen in muscle tissue). Then, glucose is released from the liver. At this point, people who do not have diabetes have a sharp drop in their insulin levels and a rise in their epinephrine (or adrenaline) levels. This triggers fat stores to release fatty acids, another fuel source. If exercise continues, muscles use more and more fatty acids for fuel; by 40 minutes or so, fatty acids account for 35% of the fuel used by muscles, and by four hours, they account for 70%.

WHEN STARTING TO EXERCISE, ALWAYS THINK ABOUT . . .

- The type, intensity, and duration of your activity
- Your starting glucose level
- Your starting basal rate
- When you took your last bolus (to know how much active insulin is present)
- The last time you had food
- The time of day
- Where your infusion set is placed on your body
- Your hydration level

In someone with diabetes, if insulin levels do not decrease, glucose and fatty acids are not released from the body's stores. Hypoglycemia will be a big risk. Even after exercise, muscles continue to use up glucose, stores are not replenished, and muscles are more sensitive to insulin, so hypoglycemia is still a risk.

In addition, you need to follow your glucose levels, determine your carbohydrate intake, and adjust your insulin levels while you are active and after you are done. If your infusion set is placed in your leg or arm and you do not have a lot of tissue there, your cannula may be closer to your muscles, resulting in your insulin being absorbed faster than if it were in a more fatty location (like your abdomen). You may notice that you are more prone to hypoglycemia during exercise if your set is in a muscular area.

GLUCOSE LEVELS BEFORE, DURING, AND AFTER EXERCISE

Before you exercise, you need to check your glucose level.

Starting with Low Glucose
If your glucose level is low (less then 70 mg/dL), then you need to correct it by ingesting carbohydrate before you begin exercising. You will need 15–30 grams of carbohydrate. Wait 15 minutes, and then check your glucose level again. You might not want to start exercis-

ing until your glucose is more than 100 mg/dL. You might also want to consider decreasing your basal insulin during exercise. It is important to check your glucose levels at least every 30–60 minutes. If there is a downward trend, you will need to ingest some carbohydrate to avoid hypoglycemia.

Quick-acting or simple carbohydrates are the best for elevating your glucose level. Glucose tabs, glucose gels, icing, juice, or a sports drink are all rapidly absorbed and good choices for quick boosts during exercise. They are also better options than solid foods that contain carbohydrate, such as snack bars, fruit, breads, crackers, or protein, because glucose raises blood glucose faster. Solid foods are better for sustaining glucose levels over long periods of exercise.

Starting in Target
If your glucose level is in the target range before you begin your activity, then you should follow your usual exercise routine in terms of duration and intensity.

Starting with High Glucose
If your glucose is more than 250 mg/dL, then you need to check for ketones before starting exercise. You should not exercise when you have ketones because of the risk of DKA. A high glucose level indicates a lack of insulin or insulin effect, and activity can cause your liver to release stored glucose and cause your blood glucose to climb even higher. Physical activity can lead your body to begin burning fat, which leads to ketone formation. If your glucose is between 250 and 300 mg/dL, you don't have ketones, and you decide to continue with your activity, then be very cautious. Take a correction bolus first (it should probably be smaller than the actual bolus calculated by your pump; this is covered later in this chapter), and check your glucose every 30–60 minutes to make sure your level is improving.

REMEMBER! IT IS NOT SAFE TO EXERCISE WITH KETONES!

Low Glucose Levels during and after Exercise

You should plan on checking glucose levels every 30–60 minutes while you exercise. Your exercise intensity and duration and your starting glucose level will give you an idea of how frequently you will need to check. If your glucose level is decreasing, you can decrease or stop your basal insulin by using the temporary basal rate or suspend feature on your pump. You can also ingest carbohydrate or do both: change your insulin dose and take carbs.

You need to check your glucose level after you are finished with activity and more frequently through the rest of the day and night. You can anticipate that glucose levels might be low after exercise (even hours later). You can help prevent or treat lows by using temporary basal rates, temporarily suspending basal insulin (if you continue to get low), or consuming extra carbohydrate without covering it with a bolus. If you do give a bolus, decrease the insulin dose so that it does not completely cover all of the carbohydrates.

Hyperglycemia after Exercise

You might find that your glucose level is high during or after exercise, perhaps much higher than when you started. Elevated glucose at these times is due to the release of epinephrine (also called adrenaline) and other hormones that help release stored glucose. Intense workouts, such as sprints or weight training, can cause a surge of adrenaline and these other hormones. You should avoid taking a correction dose of insulin during your workout, because as exercise continues high blood glucose levels often drop and can actually turn into low blood glucose levels. However, if you have decreased your basal rate, you might want to return to your usual level if hyperglycemia persists for over one hour. If your glucose is very high, you might want to consider taking a small correction dosage.

After you have completed your workout, if your blood glucose levels are still high and stay that way for over one to two hours, you should consider taking a correction bolus, but reduce it by 50%. If you continue to have hyperglycemia, you might consider a 75–100% correction bolus after another two to three hours.

ADJUST YOUR INSULIN

You usually need to reduce your basal rate when you exercise. Again, depending on the length and the intensity, you might reduce your basal insulin before, during, and after exercise or even suspend basal insulin altogether. Depending on the intensity and duration of the physical activity, you might also need to reduce the boluses you give for your meal before exercise and for the extra carbohydrate you eat before, during, and after exercise. Some of those carbs may be taken without administering insulin at all. Compared to MDI, making these adjustments is much easier with an insulin pump.

The most common way to help prevent hypoglycemia is to reduce the amount of insulin you receive in both your basal rates and your boluses (for both food and correction). Even if you disconnect your pump for contact sports or water activities, you must have some amount of active insulin. So how do you do this? Some of it is trial and error, but there are some overall principles of how to start.

Exercise and Basal Rates

Here are some tips on getting started with adjusting your basal insulin levels for exercise. Remember, your basal rate will need to be adjusted depending on the duration and intensity of the physical activity.

- **Mild activity.** You might need something like a 5–25% reduction (75–95% of your regular rate) if you are doing mild exercise, such as gardening or washing the car.

- **Moderate activity.** For any activity that makes you sweat after about 10 minutes or makes you breathe harder, you may need a 25–50% reduction in basal rates (75–50% of your regular rate).

- **High-intensity activity.** If you plan on high-intensity exercise, a 50–100% reduction or complete disconnection from the pump may be needed. Try different basal reductions. Check your glucose often.

- **Downward trends.** If your glucose tends to head downward during exercise, then you should consider another 25–50% reduction in your basal rate while exercising.

KNOW YOUR INTENSITY LEVEL

➡ Low: You can talk and sing. You don't sweat, and you have no trouble breathing.

➡ Moderate: Your breathing is harder, and you can no longer sing, although you can talk.

➡ High: No singing or talking. You begin to sweat very soon after starting the activity.

- **Zero basal rate.** If you want to eliminate basal insulin delivery altogether, you can either disconnect your pump or keep it on with a temporary basal rate of 0% for the duration of the exercise. By using a basal rate and keeping your pump connected, there is no chance that you will forget to reconnect when you are done exercising. Don't forget that if your activity lasts longer than an hour, then you need to check your glucose and determine whether you need to take a dose of insulin to replace your lost basal rate.

- **Amount of time.** The amount of time you plan on exercising might also affect your basal rate reduction. If you plan on doing short, intense workouts, then a complete reduction or disconnection of the pump is a good place to start. If you plan on doing long, strenuous, or continuous exercise (such as running or jogging, all-day hikes, or all-day sport competitions), then a very small basal rate, such as a 20% basal (80% reduction), might be a good idea. With this type of long-term activity and continued insulin delivery it is important to eat snacks along the way to keep ingesting carbohydrates. Drinking sports drinks with carbohydrates as well as water throughout will help you stay hydrated and give you glucose.

- **Your exercise pattern.** If you are someone who exercises frequently and/or for long periods of time, you may not need as drastic a decrease in your basal rates, particularly for mild exercise. Your body may already be accustomed to this type of exercise and significant reductions might cause hyperglycemia.

- **Start basal reduction before exercise.** Depending on the type, intensity, and duration of your exercise, you might want to start reducing basal insulin rates 30–60 minutes before you begin activity. This will enable you to start exercising with a reduced level of insulin in your bloodstream, which helps prevent hypoglycemia.

- **Delayed hypoglycemia and basal reduction.** Exercise may cause delayed hypoglycemia. This is especially a concern if you exercise in the afternoon, which might increase your risk of hypoglycemia during the night. Using temporary basal rates through the night can help reduce the risk of hypoglycemia. For example, you might consider a basal rate reduction of about 20% for the hours of 10:00 P.M. to 6:00 A.M. (this means you will be given 80% of your usual basal rate). Once this temporary rate is in place, wake up once or twice during the night and check your glucose levels to see if the reduction is working.

  Delayed hypoglycemia is also common after long, strenuous workouts, like hiking, marathons, or anything that lasts two or more hours. If you are doing a long stretch of exercise, you might also consider decreasing your basal rates as soon as you stop being active. A 20% reduction in basal rates for two to three hours after you finish might also reduce the risk of hypoglycemia.

- **Separate basal pattern.** If you are part of a sports team or do the same type of exercise routinely every day, a new basal pattern is probably a good idea. Switching to this "exercise" pattern for the days you plan on being active gives you consistency, convenience, and freedom.

Correction Doses and Exercise

Depending on what your glucose level is before you begin activity, and what you plan on doing and for how long, you will need to adjust how much insulin you give to correct a glucose level above your target range. You might consider a 50–100% reduction (a 100% reduction means no insulin at all). In general, for mild exercise that doesn't last very long (e.g., mowing the lawn or a leisurely walk around a park), if your starting glucose is above 180 mg/dL, then you might not need a reduction, or might only need a small one (about a 25% reduction). If you plan on doing more moderate exercise or for longer periods of time, and your glucose is 100–180 mg/dL, a 50–75% reduction is a good idea. The table below shows some guidelines for how to correct a glucose level that is above target.

Food Boluses

You often need to ingest carbohydrate before you exercise, while you are exercising (if it is of long duration), and after you are done. You decide what amount, frequency, and kind of carbohydrate to eat depending on the length and intensity of the exercise and how you feel after eating different foods, such as snack bars and drinks. Some of this you will have to learn through trial and error.

Reducing basal and bolus amounts may not be enough to prevent hypoglycemia during exercise. Many people must also eat before or during activity or both to keep their blood glucose up, so they start with a 50% reduction in food boluses.

Generally, people start with about 15 grams of carbohydrate from a liquid source, such as sports drinks, juice, or even milk (which has protein too), before starting their activity. These liquid carbs can last for about 30 minutes of moderate exercise and hit the bloodstream faster than carbohydrates from solid food and protein. Solid foods and foods that contain protein are absorbed more slowly and can help keep glucose levels elevated longer. If you are planning on doing a short amount of exercise, such as 30 minutes or less, and you have a blood glucose level within target (around 120 mg/dL), then you can

Duration (in minutes)	Intensity	Blood glucose level (mg/dL)	Possible decrease in bolus (% decrease)
<30	Mild	≥180*	50
		100–180	50–75
30–60	Moderate	≥180*	50–75
		100–180	75–100
≥60	Intense	≥180*	50–85
		100–180	85–100

*If your blood glucose level is above 250 mg/dL and you have ketones, DO NOT EXERCISE.

drink 15 grams of carbohydrate and you may not need to take any insulin. If you plan on doing more sustained exercise, such as an hour or more, then you may need to eat solid carbohydrates too. This might include a half sandwich (or whole sandwich, depending on what the activity is) with protein, such as meat or cheese. If you cannot exercise with a full stomach, eat your meal about 30–45 minutes before exercising so you have time to digest, and then reduce your bolus according to the planned duration and intensity of your activity.

Treating Lows during and after Exercise

Even if you have reduced your basal rates and correction boluses and have eaten, hypoglycemia still happens. Treating it may need to be a little more vigorous than the usual 15 grams of carbohydrate that you normally take for an everyday low. Thirty grams of carbohydrate may need to be eaten first and 15 grams more if you plan on doing more intense exercise after you recover. *It is important that you do not continue to exercise if your blood glucose levels have not increased.* After eating, wait 15 minutes and then test again. If you still have not seen a rise in your blood glucose, eat 15 grams of carbohydrate and wait another 15 minutes. Be sure to always have snacks and quick-acting carbs handy (e.g., glucose tabs or juice) when you exercise!

A FEW FINAL THOUGHTS

- Safety is essential when it comes to exercise. Be prepared for hypoglycemia and hyperglycemia. Tell people around you what to do and how to help you in case of an emergency. If you are part of a sports team, inform your coach or some close teammates about what to do if you are unable to treat yourself. Let them know where your supplies are and how to administer them.

- Drink plenty of water! Dehydration can increase the chance of ketones and make it harder to get rid of them if they develop. A healthy body is a hydrated body. You may need to drink carbohydrates during your workout to keep your glucose in the target range.

- If you are exercising outside on a hot day, bring a cooler to put your pump and supplies in so that they don't overheat in the sun. If insulin gets too hot, it can lose its effectiveness. Intense heat may also damage your pump! If this happens and you don't have a back-up insulin source, you are likely to develop high blood glucose levels and can potentially develop ketones. Always have a plan for your activity that includes backup insulin and plenty of glucose/snacks.

CHAPTER REVIEW

➡ Hypoglycemia is a risk of exercise. The more you exercise, the more sensitive to insulin you will become. Being more sensitive to insulin means you might need to take less insulin overall. And not just while you are exercising, but hours later and in the night.

➡ When you start to exercise, you always need to think about the following: the type, intensity, and duration of your activity; your starting glucose; your starting basal rate; when you took your last bolus (so you know how much active insulin is in your body); the last time you ate or had carbs; the time of day; where your infusion set is placed on your body; and your hydration level. Do not exercise if you have ketones.

➡ Check your glucose level every 30–60 minutes while you exercise. The more intense the exercise is, the longer its duration, and the lower your starting glucose, the more often you need to check. Treat low glucose levels. You need to measure your glucose level after you are done being active and more frequently through the rest of the day and night. You can anticipate that glucose levels might be low even hours after exercise. Be aware that you might find your glucose level is high during or after exercise, possibly much higher than when you started. Elevated glucose at these times is due to the release of epinephrine (adrenaline). You may not want to treat this high immediately, because exercise can still cause your levels to drop later.

➡ Ways to treat hypoglycemia associated with exercise include using temporary basal rates, temporarily suspending basal insulin if you continue to get low glucose levels, or ingesting extra carbohydrate without bolusing. If you do give a bolus, decrease the amount of insulin you take to cover your carbohydrate intake.

IN THIS CHAPTER

➡ Types of Infusion Sets

➡ Tubing Length

➡ Site Rotation and Placement of Infusion Set and Pump

➡ Troubleshooting Issues at the Insertion Site

CHAPTER 8

THE FACTS ABOUT INFUSION SETS

There are many factors that influence which infusion set you will use when you first start the pump. You may want to see and use different infusion sets to determine which one or ones work best for you. Your choices may depend on your lifestyle and body type. (Don't forget, patch pumps do not have infusion sets.)

An infusion set consists of several components.

- **Tubing.** The tubing attaches to the insulin reservoir. One end is inserted into the insulin pump and the other end is affixed to the insertion site itself.

- **Infusion sets and cannulas (or needles).** At the opposite end of the reservoir is the part of the infusion set that attaches to your body. It consists of an adhesive tape and the catheter or cannula, which is a small tube that sits under the skin in the subcutaneous

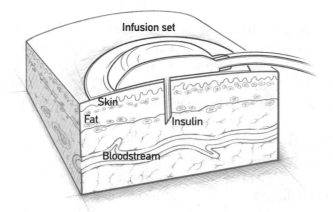

fat (the fat under the skin). Through this very small tube or needle, the insulin is delivered to your body.

- **Detachable section.** There is a small platform where the cannula connects to the tubing and a section that is detachable so that the insulin pump and tubing can be removed for activities, bathing, or other reasons. In some cases, the tubing disconnects from the infusion site near the base, and in other cases there are a couple of inches of tubing and then a disconnect area.

For the most part, infusion sets are the same, but there are some important details that distinguish one from another and may help or hinder your diabetes care. Let's first start out with the two major categories of sets: Teflon® and metal catheters.

TYPES OF INFUSION SETS

Teflon® Catheters

Teflon® catheters are made of a flexible plastic material that makes them comfortable. The flexibility allows the catheter to move with you but it also can get kinked or bent while still under the skin. When this happens, insulin delivery can be slowed or stopped, potentially leading to high glucose levels. The cannula in a Teflon® set comes in angles of 90° and 30°.

90° Angle
A 90°-angle infusion set is inserted straight into the body and lies perpendicular to your skin. It can be used in any fatty area because there will be enough space between the tip of the cannula and muscle. If it is too close to the muscle, insulin absorption can be affected and sites can be more prone to kinking. For people with more fat under the skin, there is a 9-mm cannula. For leaner people and children with less body fat, there is a 6-mm cannula. Choosing a cannula length short enough to avoid muscle but also long enough to decrease the risk of it coming out (this can be an issue with the 6-mm cannula) is important for complete and uninterrupted insulin delivery.

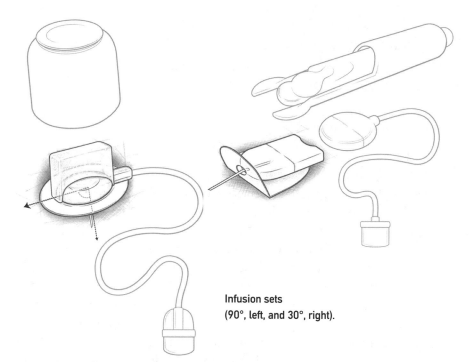

Infusion sets
(90°, left, and 30°, right).

A HANDY RULE

A good rule to think about when choosing which set to put where is if you can pinch up at least 3/4 inch or about 2 cm of fat at the site, then you can use a 90° set. However, when inserting the 90° set, it is not a good idea to pinch up the tissue. These 90° sets work very well in areas that are hard to reach (such as the arm, buttock, or hip) and are fleshier, or are good for people who are wary or scared of needles because there is less visibility of the needle and catheter itself. Leaner people with less body fat tend to have more problems with the 90° sets kinking or pulling free, so they might find that a 30° infusion set is a better choice.

SOMETHING TO THINK ABOUT!

Many people use both 90° and 30° sets on different areas of their body, depending on the amount of fat at each site.

30° Angle
A 30°-angle infusion set is inserted at an angle of about 30°. Because of its angled application, these sets are good for very lean or slender people without a lot of body fat. The 30° sets have a longer cannula than the 90° sets—up to 12–13 mm. These sets can be a little intimidating at first. When inserted correctly, these infusion sets avoid hitting muscle. To correctly insert this type of set, insert it at a 30° angle. If this cannula is inserted into the abdomen, the set must be inserted horizontally. Because of the angle and longer cannula, these sets tend to have fewer problems with kinking and pulling out, especially during exercise. It is harder to insert 30° sets in areas other than the abdominal area, but it's not impossible.

Metal Infusion Sets
Metal infusion sets, unlike the Teflon® sets, have a cannula that is made of metal. They are only inserted at a 90° angle. They generally are worn with the same level of comfort as the flexible cannula. These sets are good for people who have problems with kinking or cannulas popping out. These sets have a disconnection area that is about 4 inches from the site and adhesive tape along the tubing.

Infusion Set Insertion
Infusion sets can be inserted manually or with an injector device, and some sets come with their own built-in injectors that are disposed of individually. Insertion devices can sometimes help with pain or fear of the needle as they make the process smooth and quick. The injector devices make a clicking sound that can be intimidating for some people.

With the 30° sets, there is a small "window" area in the adhesive tape that shows where the catheter is inserted into the skin. For people who have issues with their sets falling out, this can be a useful feature because you can periodically and easily check the status or condition of your site. You can also see if there is any puffiness, redness, or other signs of a problem at the insertion site. There is no viewing window with a 90° infusion set, so the actual insertion area is less visible. A catheter on a 90° infusion set can come out without you recognizing that it has pulled away.

Inserting the 30° set manually can help people fine-tune the angle that works best for them. For both set angles, manual insertion gives the person a degree of control over pacing and placement that can't be mimicked with the insertion devices.

TUBING LENGTH

There are several lengths of tubing to connect the infusion set on the body to the reservoir in the pump. Generally, there is a shorter length (around 23–24 inches) and a longer length (about 40 inches). If the tubing length is too short, it can pull at the site and loosen the tape, leading to a kinked or removed cannula. If the tubing is too long, it has the tendency to get caught on things like doorknobs, dressers, and corners, and even on other people! Taller people tend to feel more comfortable with longer tubing, although this is not always the case.

Considerations for Tube Selection
Think about where you want to wear your pump. This should be the first thing to consider when determining your tubing length. Here are some other good questions to ask yourself before you choose your tubing length:

- Where will your pump be when you're sleeping? Do you want to keep it attached to you? Are you a restless sleeper or can you place your pump on your bedside table or under your pillow? Do you want to place your attached pump next to you on the bed?

A longer tubing length can be more convenient for people who want to place it next to them in bed or under a pillow.

- Most people connect their pumps to their pants. Think about when you go to the bathroom and your pants are on the floor. When you stand up, is your tubing going to be long enough that it won't pull out your infusion set?

- When you change your clothing, do you need to place your pump on a nearby object, such as a dresser or bed? How close do you want to stand next to such objects?

- Some women place their pumps in carriers in their bras or on the side of their thigh under skirts or dresses. What length of tubing might this require to reach from your infusion set comfortably?

- What will you do with the extra tubing? If you prefer the longer tubing, you need to manage the excess, so it does not get caught on other things or get pulled out of your body. There are companies that make devices that roll up tubing, or you can coil it yourself and place a piece of tape around it. Just make sure that whatever approach you take, you can easily undo it so you don't accidently pull on your set when you move your pump.

As opposed to catheter length and type, tubing length is determined by personal preference, so if you don't like the tubing length you originally chose, it's not a problem. There is plenty of variety. Tubing length is something that might also change for different activities. Keep a few different lengths on hand just in case a situation arises in which you will need longer or shorter tubing.

SITE ROTATION AND PLACEMENT OF INFUSION SET AND PUMP

It is important to understand that an infusion set is in place for two to three days straight. The insulin infusion and the constant presence of the catheter can cause irritation and the development of fatty lumps and scar tissue. If this occurs, absorption of insulin at that site may not be as effective. This is why site rotation is encouraged.

Creating a site-rotation plan helps eliminate the overuse or accidental reuse of a site. Some people create templates where they can record when a site was last used. Other people follow a circular rotation pattern and alternate from side to side. Your rotational preference is personal and can be changed, but make sure that you do not use the same place each time!

Where to Place Your Infusion Set

Infusion sets can be put into any area if there is enough fatty tissue to keep the cannula from pushing into muscle. Most people have some fleshy areas around their abdomen and on their buttocks. Even very thin people generally have enough tissue in these areas to successfully use an infusion set. Any 90° set can be used if there is about 3/4 inch of fat when you pinch; a 30° set takes about 1/2 inch. Your diabetes team can help you find your best places. The most common areas for site rotation are the abdomen, buttocks, upper thigh, and back of the arm.

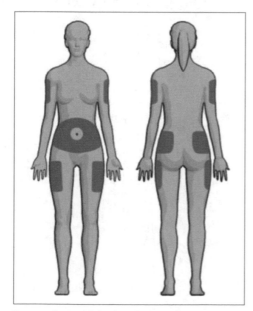

Commonly used injection sites.

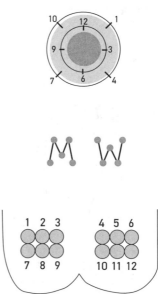

Three methods of site rotation.

The abdomen is the most frequently used site. Most people can use a large area of their abdomen, both above and below the waistline. Insulin is absorbed the best in this area, so it is also recommended by health care professionals. If you decide to try this area, make sure that the waistband of your clothing doesn't rub against the infusion set. The stomach area also offers the advantages of good visibility and easy access.

The buttock is also very popular, particularly with young children—it is out of site and out of reach. Almost everyone has enough padding there, and a good twist around or a mirror can lead to a successful insertion. If you're wary of sitting on the infusion site, have no fear! There is plenty of space above where you actually sit that can be used for the infusion set.

The upper leg can be used, but there is more potential for hitting muscle. If you insert directly into muscle, it might be painful. In addition, it might increase the rate of absorption and cause low glucose levels.

When the back of the arm is used, the tubing must climb through your shirt and sleeves and find its way to your pump, wherever it is you intend to place it.

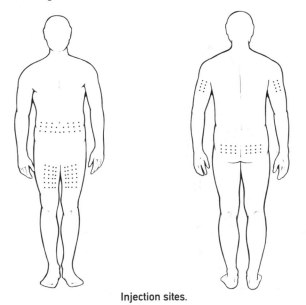

Injection sites.

Where to Place Your Pump

Where you clip, hang, bag, or store your insulin pump is up to you (unless you're using a patch pump). There are some common ways to carry it and some rather creative ways to deal with its constant presence.

It is easiest to wear the pump around your waist. You can put it in your pocket or clip it onto your belt or waistband (pumps come with clips and holders). In addition, you can buy pouches and cases with belt loops and clips. Some children need to be kept away from their pumps, so harnesses and pouches are good options (these also keep it away from curious classmates and friends who might want to press buttons). If you keep your pump in your front pocket (this is often more possible for men with looser pants), then you might think about clipping a small hole in the inside of the pocket, so you can feed your tubing through the hole—the tubing will have less opportunity to get caught on something. When wearing skirts or dresses without pockets or waistbands, some women use pouches and similar devices to strap their pumps to the inside of their thighs (like garters with a pouch) or they clip them to their bras.

There are other situations when you will have to deal with the placement of your pump that might not occur to you until you encounter them, but below are a few to think about.

Sleeping

If you are a restless sleeper, it might be a good idea to find a way to fix the pump comfortably to your pajamas. Or try placing it under your pillow (but be aware that you might not hear the alarms). If you sleep fairly calmly, you can put it on a bedside table or next to you in the bed. (If you have a restless partner in bed with you, then you might want to think about the possibility of him or her rolling over it as well).

Many people worry about rolling over their infusion site, tubing, and pump while sleeping, but everything is durable and should survive the impact. You shouldn't be able to feel the infusion site when you roll onto it (if there is tenderness or pain, then there might be something wrong with the site and a site rotation might be necessary). Tubing shouldn't kink, and it takes a significant amount of direct pressure to the buttons to activate them. The amount of pressure from your body is spread out when you are lying down and there is plenty of give in your mattress to avoid any kinking or unwanted pump-button activation.

Exercise

Most pumps are fairly sturdy and water resistant, so you can wear one during exercise—regardless of sweating. A number of protective hard cases are available if you don't want to remove your pump during rougher sports (such cases are highly recommended). Also, activities that involve water (e.g., swimming, scuba diving, snorkeling, water skiing, tubing, surfing) require you to disconnect the pump. Most pumps are water resistant and can get wet, but be cautious when submerging them in water. Even if the pump is designed to be water resistant, if there is any small crack in the casing, this could ruin your pump or cause a dangerous malfunction.

When you disconnect from the pump, the cannula is left inserted into your body and the tubing and pump are removed. Often sets will come with clips or coverings to keep the site clean and free of things like sand. The sets are designed so only insulin is allowed into your body, so don't worry about swimming with a disconnected set. When you disconnect for sports and exercise, it is important to watch your blood glucose carefully and to periodically reconnect to give a small amount of insulin to counteract the loss of your basal insulin.

Intimacy

When you are engaged in intimate activities, pumps can easily be disconnected and put away. It might be a good idea to suspend your pump's functions during this time because many pumps will sound an alarm to remind you that it has been suspended. This alarm will notify you if you happen to fall asleep without reconnecting.

Showers and Baths

You should disconnect from the pump for showers and baths. Remember to reconnect after you are done. Some pumps are water resistant and can be worn.

TROUBLESHOOTING ISSUES AT THE INSERTION SITE

Here are some common issues that you might experience with your infusion sets:

- **Irritation from the tape.** Some people have issues with the adhesive on the tapes irritating their skin, lasting too long, or coming off early. Although allergies and sensitivities are uncommon, they do unfortunately happen. Some people experience a rash after removing the tape or while the set is inserted into the area. There are several wipes that can add a level of protection between the skin and the adhesive. If that is not enough, inserting the set through a dressing also helps completely separate the irritant from the skin.

- **Adhesive on the skin.** If you have problems with tape staying on (this is very common), there are several wipes that will help with adhesion. It is important to always start by wiping the intended area with alcohol. This helps remove bacteria and surface oils, which can impede the stickiness of the tape (on the note of bacteria, don't blow on your site to dry it because this can introduce germs to the area and increase the chances of getting an infection). If you need even more assistance with getting the tape to stay attached to your skin, you can try more potent preparations. The only problem with some of these potent wipes is removing the set later. People who sweat a lot or exercise frequently might also try placing another piece of tape over the top of the set. You might also think about putting a piece of tape about 2 inches above the site for added security in case tubing is caught on something. Doing this is especially helpful if you have trouble with the set sticking in place.

  If you have a problem with removal, then there are products that can help with that too (they've thought of everything!). All of these products can be applied to the top of the tape and then left for a few minutes to sink in and start to dissolve the stickiness underneath. Then as you slowly remove the tape, wipe the solvent under the tape to detach the rest of it. Just make sure you wash off the solvent completely or your next set might not stick very well!

- **Bubbles in tubing.** Several things can cause bubbles to appear in your tubing, and it is important to regularly check for these because an inch of air in the tubing can be equivalent to 0.50 unit of insulin! For many people, that can be a significant amount of their basal rate and can cause a high glucose level. Bubbles can form from insulin going from cold to room temperature (this applies to people who take their insulin bottles right from the refrigerator). If you can, try to let your insulin warm up a little bit before filling your reservoir and before changing your set. A change in altitude, such as when flying in an airplane or driving into the mountains, can increase bubble frequency.

  Bubbles can be removed by a Fill or Prime function. The pump records this amount of insulin but does not count it toward a meal or correction bolus, so the pump won't think that there is active insulin. Make sure you disconnect before you prime to remove bubbles, or you might receive extra insulin that you don't need. It's a worthwhile habit to check for bubbles in the morning and before you go to bed. Bubbles, other than keeping you from receiving insulin, will not harm you if they enter your body.

- **Pain.** If your set is painful, it might be a sign of infection or that you have inserted your cannula too close to muscle. In either case, it will be a good idea to change your set because insulin absorption will be affected and will be absorbed faster or not at all, depending on what's wrong. If there is any puffiness, redness, swelling, discharge, or warmth at your set, you should change your set and then monitor your glucose levels as well as your body temperature. If you develop a fever, it could mean that you have an infection, and you should not only change your set immediately but also contact your health care team or your primary care physician. Without a fever, it is most likely okay to just change your set. However, if you have a painful, red, hot lump—which might contain bacteria and pus—that gets worse or won't go away, you should contact your health care team.

- **High blood glucose after a set change.** If your blood glucose level increases (without an obvious cause) after a set change, you might have forgotten to prime or fill your cannula. This prime is different from the prime or fill that fills the tubing with insulin, because the cannula cannot be filled until after the needle (in the case of the Teflon® sets) has been removed after an insertion.

Infusion sets operate best when kept in for two to three days. After this, the absorbability of the site itself diminishes. Some people see an increase in insulin resistance on or after that third day. Also, if a set is left in too long, the risk of infection increases, and you certainly don't want that!

Taking proper care of your site by cleaning it thoroughly before insertion, checking regularly for bubbles, and changing it on time will help prevent highs and infections from happening.

CHAPTER REVIEW

➡ The infusion set is made up of tubing that attaches at one end to the insulin reservoir in the insulin pump. The other end affixes to the insertion site itself—the cannula or needle and the detachable section.

➡ There are several lengths of tubing to connect the infusion set on the body to the reservoir in the pump. Determining the correct length for you (from 23–24 inches to about 40 inches) is important.

➡ It is important to understand that an infusion set is in place for two to three days straight. Local insulin infusion and the constant presence of the catheter can cause irritation and the development of fatty lumps and scar tissue. If this occurs, absorption of insulin at that site may not work as expected. This is why site rotation is encouraged.

➡ Issues that occur, such as irritation at the insertion site, residual adhesive on the skin, bubbles in the tubing, pain at the insertion site, and high glucose levels after insertion, require troubleshooting.

CHAPTER 9

SPECIAL CIRCUMSTANCES
SICK DAYS, IN-HOSPITAL USE, DISCONTINUING PUMP THERAPY

Paying attention to your diabetes when you're sick or in need of hospitalization is always important. It is no less important when you're on insulin pump therapy. In fact, in many ways, it may be easier. With an insulin pump and meticulous glucose monitoring, you can quickly make changes in insulin delivery to avoid episodes of hypoglycemia and hyperglycemia that could complicate your illness or delay your recovery.

SICK DAYS

When you have diabetes, an illness can make your blood glucose control difficult. When your body is stressed by illness, particularly when you are vomiting, have diarrhea, or have a fever, your body releases hormones (counterregulatory hormones) that order your liver to release stored glucose and tell your fat to release free fatty acids to form ketones. Your body does this when you're sick because you need more energy to fight off infection and to repair damaged tissue. If you don't have diabetes, your body releases more insulin to control the rise in glucose and ketones. When you have diabetes, you need to manage the process on your own, by monitoring your glucose and ketone levels and by increasing insulin delivery to manage the situation. In addition, you are at risk of hypoglycemia when you are ill, particularly if you don't eat or drink, are vomiting, or have diarrhea. Either way, if you don't control glucose and ketones, you can end up developing DKA. This can make you much sicker, potentially requiring a prolonged hospitalization, and delay your recovery.

CATEGORIES OF ILLNESS

Illnesses are broken down into two categories:

1. illnesses that can potentially lead to dehydration and are accompanied by lack of appetite, nausea, vomiting, or diarrhea.

2. illnesses that don't increase the risk of dehydration, such as colds.

Illnesses with Risk of Dehydration

Dehydrating illnesses can be more dangerous if you have diabetes. They require more attention and possibly a call or visit to your health care team. In this group are illnesses that lead to reduced intake of fluids (fluids are more important than food), nausea, vomiting, or diarrhea. If your blood glucose is going low or already low because of such an illness, temporarily reduce your basal rate by 25–50%. If you need to suspend insulin delivery, don't suspend it for more than 30 minutes or you will increase the risk of developing ketones. If hypoglycemia continues, you might consider administering a low dose of glucagon, but before you do this you will need to discuss this approach with your health care team.

If your glucose level is high, you must maintain a balance between increasing insulin delivery and maintaining hydration, remembering that if your glucose level is above 180–200 mg/dL, then you will likely urinate more often because of the glucose being excreted in your urine. A temporary basal rate with a 25–50% increase or a small cor-

LOW-DOSE OR MINI-DOSE GLUCAGON

DOSE:

- 2 units for children aged 2 years or younger
- 1 unit per year of age for children aged 3–15 years
- 15 units for children older than 15 years

Raises the glucose level 50–200 mg/dL in around 30 minutes.

rection bolus (but less than what is calculated by the pump's bolus calculator) may be enough to bring your blood glucose level back down into your target range. You don't want to bring the glucose too low, however, because you could develop hypoglycemia. This is especially a problem if you are unable to keep down fluids, which would make it very difficult to treat a low.

Illnesses that Don't Increase Risk of Dehydration

This category of illnesses is less worrisome, and the goal is to get your glucose level to just below the upper range of your target, avoiding both hyperglycemia and hypoglycemia. Don't focus on food—fluids are more important.

Sick-Day Treatments

The basic treatments for sick days on the pump are very similar to what you did before on MDI. Below are some key things to keep in mind.

Start a Log
Keep track of the following:

- glucose levels

- ketones

- temperature

- oral intake of fluids with carbohydrate/glucose (count grams of carbohydrate/glucose ingested)

- oral intake of fluids without carbohydrate/glucose (fluids are important for maintaining hydration)

- urination

- episodes of vomiting or diarrhea

Check Your Glucose Level Often
Follow your glucose levels very closely, every one to two hours. You might need to check every 30 minutes if your glucose levels are changing rapidly. If you are using a CGM, look at the trend and abso-

lute value every 10–15 minutes. The goal is to keep your blood glucose at the upper level of your target range and to avoid hypoglycemia and hyperglycemia.

Stay Hydrated by Drinking Fluids
It's easy to become dehydrated when you're sick. Dehydration results from vomiting, diarrhea, and hyperglycemia. If your glucose level is above 180–200 mg/dL, you will urinate more often as your body tries to flush out the extra glucose through your urine. After vomiting, wait 30–60 minutes, and then start hydrating yourself with teaspoons of water, progressing to tablespoons, and then to ounces. When your glucose level is below 150 mg/dL, treat it with glucose-containing fluids, such as sports drinks, electrolyte-containing liquids, or flat sugar-containing sodas without caffeine. The goal is to try to retain 4–6 ounces of fluids (2–4 ounces for younger children) every 30–60 minutes until you are rehydrated.

Continue to Take Your Insulin
This is very important. Your body still needs insulin in order to use the sugar in your blood for energy, and you need all the energy you can get when you are sick. Even if you are not eating or drinking fluids with carbohydrate, you still need insulin. You might even need more insulin because the stress hormones released in response to illness can cause blood glucose levels to increase.

Check Ketones at the Beginning of and Periodically during Your Illness
When you're sick, your body may start to break down fat for energy. When this happens, ketones are produced. This may happen even if your blood glucose isn't high. If ketones are present, check every time you urinate or every four hours if you are monitoring ketones in blood. If they are not present, check for them two times a day until you are well. If you become nauseated or begin vomiting, check again; these can be signs of the presence of ketones. It is very important to know if ketones are present because this means you need more fluid, more insulin, and more glucose if your blood glucose level is below 150–200 mg/dL.

Check Your Pump Site and Tubing
Changing your set when you become sick is a good idea so you know that your site is working, your site absorption is adequate, and your cannula is not kinked or bent. By starting out with a fresh site, you have a better chance of having your insulin absorbed correctly when you need it most. If you just changed your set, look for bubbles and maybe add some extra tape for security.

Let Others Know What to Do When You Are Ill
If you become too sick to check your glucose and manage your diabetes, you need help. Help can come in three ways:

1. Someone who has been taught (your spouse, best friend, roommate, parents, etc.) how to check your glucose, deliver insulin via your pump, administer glucagon, and more. In other words, someone else knows how to manage your diabetes, and they are prepared to help you while you are ill.

2. Someone who knows how to check and interpret your glucose levels, give you glucose orally, and when to call for help.

3. Someone who knows how to call for help, either from your diabetes team or 911.

The more people who can help you manage your diabetes, the safer you will be during an illness or accident.

Your Glucose Level and Some Medications

Some medications, such as inhalers for asthma or steroid-based pain medications, might increase your glucose level. Before taking medications, discuss the effect the medication might have on your diabetes management with your health care team. If a certain medication

> **A GOOD IDEA**
> It is a good idea to teach someone how to disconnect or suspend your pump if you develop severe hypoglycemia and are unable to treat yourself.

is known to increase glucose levels, discuss whether you should increase your basal rates or just rely on correction doses. Some medications also contain sugar for flavoring. Sugared cough drops can have up to 5 grams of carbohydrate per lozenge! Take the necessary amount of insulin for these types of medications, and as always, test often and record what you find.

TROUBLESHOOTING HIGH AND LOW GLUCOSE LEVELS

You should develop a routine to troubleshoot high glucose levels. This includes checking your infusion site, the infusion set tubing, the connection between your reservoir and infusion set, the reservoir itself, the effectiveness of your insulin (is it expired or has it been exposed to excessive cold or heat?), and the insulin pump. The table on p. 117 lists what to check, what questions to ask yourself, and what to do.

In addition, you should assess your own health and well-being. Ask yourself if you feel like you are getting sick. Did you take any medications? Are you stressed? Are you about to get your period? If something is going on with your overall health status, you may want to contact your diabetes team or prepare for sick-day management.

You can also help your troubleshooting along if you know what can cause hypoglycemia and hyperglycemia when you use an insulin pump. The table on p. 118 describes many of these cases.

HYPERGLYCEMIA AND KETONES

Whenever glucose levels are above 250 mg/dL, you should check for ketones. Whether the test for ketones is positive or negative will determine how you should treat the elevated blood glucose.

Ketones are acids made up of acetoacetic acid and beta-hydroxybutyric acid and are sometimes called ketoacids. They are made when fat is broken down. Fatty acids are freed from fat, and then

Troubleshooting Guidelines

What to Check	Questions to Ask	If Yes...
Infusion site	– Is it red, irritated, or painful? – Is it wet or does it smell like insulin?	Change infusion set, reservoir, and insulin.
Infusion set tubing	– Are there bubbles (larger than champagne bubbles) in the tubing? – Is there blood in the tubing?	Change infusion set, reservoir, and insulin.
Connection between reservoir and infusion set	– Are there leaks or breaks? – Is connection loose or easily moved?	Change infusion set, reservoir, and insulin if unable to correct the problem by tightening.
Reservoir or cartridge	– Is it loaded correctly? – Is the reservoir empty? – Are there excessive bubbles?	Change infusion set, reservoir, and insulin if unable to correct the issue.
Insulin	– Has insulin vial expired? – Has insulin been exposed to high temperatures or direct sunlight?	Change infusion set and reservoir, using a new vial of insulin. (When in doubt, change it out!)
Check insulin pump settings – Bolus delivery – Basal rates – Time	– Was last meal bolus missed? – Are basal rates set incorrectly? – Is time set correctly?	– Give correction dose – Reset basal rates – Set time correctly
Insulin pump	– Is insulin pump not working or inoperable? – Not sure if insulin pump has a problem?	Call the toll-free help line for your insulin pump manufacturer. The number is often located on the pump itself.

the liver makes them into ketones. The body forms these ketones when it is trying to produce more fuel because there isn't enough energy being received from metabolized glucose and glycogen (glucose stores released from the liver). When ketones build up in your bloodstream, you have ketosis and are at risk of developing DKA, a serious and potentially life-threatening condition.

You develop ketones when you do not have enough insulin in your bloodstream. You can develop ketones, even if you take your usual dose of insulin, if the amount you took does not meet your metabolic needs at the time. This occurs with infection, stress, or

Causes of Hypoglycemia and Hyperglycemia While on an Insulin Pump

Hyperglycemia	Hypoglycemia
Too little insulin given as bolus	Too much insulin given as boluses
• Incorrect ICR for corrections	• Incorrect ICR for corrections
• Incorrect ICR for food	• Incorrect ICR for food
• Underestimating food intake	• Overestimating food intake
• Missed bolus	• Insulin stacking
• Manual bolusing	• Manual bolusing
• Delayed timing of food bolus	• Delayed eating after bolus
Basal rates have not been increased as needed	Basal rates are too high
• Basal infusion rates too low	• Need different pattern
• Need temporary increase or different pattern	• Need temporary decrease
Infusion set problems	Infusion set problems
• Cannula kinked or dislodged	• Not disconnected from body when priming or filling tubing
• Poor site with inadequate absorption	
• Inflammation or infection at the site	
• Air bubbles	
Other causes	Other causes
• Insulin expired or spoiled from heating or freezing	• Pump clock is wrong
• Pump malfunction	• Primed while attached
• Battery failure	

illness. Commonly, the body makes ketones when blood glucose levels are very high. However, you may have only mild hyperglycemia, a normal glucose level, or even a low glucose value (during starvation) and still produce ketones. Your body tries to eliminate ketones through breathing (your breathing becomes deep and labored and the ketones make your breath smell like rotting fruit) and urination (causing you also to lose important electrolytes, like potassium and sodium).

It is important for everyone using insulin pump therapy to understand that they can develop ketones if the pump stops delivering insulin. This is because there will no longer be any long-acting or basal insulin in the body. Ketones may form as quickly as three hours after

When blood glucose is ≥250 mg/dL, check for KETONES and follow these guidelines.

Positive for ketones (or if nauseated, vomiting, urinating excessively, or have fruity-smelling breath)	Negative for ketones

• Give a correction dose by injection
• Change infusion set, reservoir, and insulin
• Check blood glucose every 1–2 hours and give insulin by injection until blood glucose levels are within target range
• If the glucose level is not going down and you have moderate to high ketones, nausea, vomiting, or difficulty breathing, call your health care provider or go to the emergency room
	• Give a correction dose through the insulin pump
	• Recheck blood glucose in 1 hour
	• If blood glucose has not decreased in 1 hour
	  – give an insulin injection
	  – change infusion set, reservoir, and insulin
	• Continue to check your blood glucose until glucose levels are within the desired range

In this situation, it is best to give insulin by syringe, in case the high glucose level is caused by an issue with the pump or any of its parts.	*The most common causes of unexplained hyperglycemia that does not respond to a correction bolus include a kinked or displaced cannula, an infusion set or reservoir issue, or a "bad" vial of insulin.*

insulin interruption. If you have an infusion-set malfunction or blocked tubing or cannula, you may not realize that you are not receiving insulin. You may know only when you find a high glucose level and then check for ketones.

Urine ketones can be detected with ketone strips. A small detection patch changes color according to the level of ketones present (negative, small, moderate, large, and very large). Blood ketones can be checked with a normal fingerstick by a special machine. Readings are in millimoles per liter (mmol/L) and range from 0.0 to ≥3.0.

With ketones, extra insulin is given every two to four hours until you no longer have ketones. Insulin resistance can occur when you have ketosis (meaning that the insulin you take may be less effective), so extra insulin beyond your usual correction for high glucose may be needed. You should discuss this with your health care team, but here are some basic concepts.

➡ **Small to moderate ketones.** Calculate your correction bolus for your glucose level. Add 5–10% of your total daily insulin (you can find this in the history or utilities/daily totals section of your pump). If this is your first high glucose with ketones, you can take this bolus by pump. Recheck after one to two hours. If this is your second high glucose with ketones, take the correction and additional insulin by syringe. Then change your set, make sure your reservoir is filled, and verify that your pump is working. Continue rechecking and taking correction insulin every two to four hours until you are negative for ketones. But you do need to keep in mind the effects of active insulin.

➡ **Large ketones.** You should take your calculated insulin dose plus 10–20% of your daily insulin total by syringe. Change your set. Be sure that your reservoir is filled and your pump is working. Call your health care team and recheck both glucose and ketones after one to two hours.

➡ **DRINK FLUIDS!** The more fluids you can drink, the easier it is to help your body flush out the ketones. Drink plenty of water or glucose-free liquids when your glucose is above 180–200 mg/dL. When your glucose level falls below 180 mg/dL, if you still have ketones, start drinking glucose-containing liquids. Juice, tea with sugar or honey, flat sugar-containing sodas, or frozen pops with sugar will all work. Take insulin to cover the glucose you are ingesting.

KETONES AND HYPOGLYCEMIA

If ketones form and you have normal or low blood glucose, drink fluids that contain glucose. Don't take bolus insulin until your glucose level is high enough to require correction.

HOSPITAL VISITS

Elective Admission

If you are scheduled to go to the hospital for an elective admission, you need to discuss your insulin delivery plan with your diabetes team and the team that will care for you in the hospital before you are admitted. If you decide to remain on your insulin pump, bring extra supplies—infusion sets (and inserters), reservoirs, batteries—to last you through the number of days you will be in the hospital. Write down or copy the download of all your pump settings. During your hospitalization, you might need to increase or decrease basal rates and boluses depending on your ability to eat and move about and the level of stress or illness. Be sure the infusion set is not located in a place where you will lie on it constantly, and be sure to check the site frequently for infection or irritation.

Emergency Room Visits and Emergency Hospitalizations

It is critical that you have a medical ID bracelet or necklace that tells people you have diabetes. The health care personnel you encounter in the emergency room and hospital must pay close attention to your glucose levels. They must manage your diabetes, and one option is to continue on your insulin pump. They can retrieve your basal insulin infusion rates as well as your bolus history from your insulin pump. They can also find a history of your glucose levels in the pump or meter. These pieces of information will be helpful as they develop your diabetes treatment plan and as they consult your diabetes team.

Surgery

Insulin pumps are usually not used during surgery. You and/or a family member need to discuss your insulin delivery and glucose monitoring plans with your medical teams. You want to be sure that your glucose levels are checked often (at least every hour) before, during, and after the procedure. You might receive insulin by injection or by vein. As soon as you are able, ask about how much insulin you have and are presently receiving and about your glucose control. As much as possible, participate in your diabetes care.

Pregnancy

Insulin pump therapy is ideal during pregnancy and should be considered in the preconception period, when the goal is to intensify management, lower A1C, reduce hypoglycemia, and stabilize glucose levels in order to help create the best outcomes for the mother and the baby.

Insulin requirements change during pregnancy. In the last trimester, basal rates may need to be increased by 0.3–0.6 unit per hour and ICR may need to be increased by 50–100%. These high rates are required to reduce hyperglycemia (this is dangerous to the fetus), but they also put the pregnant woman at risk for hypoglycemia. Target glucose and A1C levels are much lower during pregnancy. Pregnant women are also at greater risk for ketone buildup and consequently, DKA. Therefore, troubleshooting highs is essential (a CGM can be a valuable addition at this time). Site selection during pregnancy can be difficult, so careful attention should be paid to the skin, particularly if infusion sets are placed in the abdomen.

Insulin pumps should be used during labor and delivery, but an infusion of insulin by vein may be required if hyperglycemia cannot be controlled. As soon as delivery occurs, basal rates need to be significantly reduced because the baby is no longer using maternal glucose.

Women should be encouraged to breast-feed. During nursing, basal rate reduction is usually required. The ability of women with type 1 diabetes to now have healthy pregnancies and babies is due to careful, attentive management of diabetes before and during pregnancy.

TIME OFF THE PUMP

There are times when you just can't wear the pump (e.g., long days of water activity) or when you decide you want a break from the pump. Those types of days when you are disconnected for only a short period of time (less than five hours) are easily regulated with periodic boluses from the pump. If you are planning on a full day off the pump or you tend to have several days off the pump, you might want to consider some of the following options.

- **Partial pump vacation (disconnecting multiple times in a day).** If you want to leave the infusion set in but only use the pump intermittently, you can take some basal insulin by injection to help reduce the risk of extreme highs or lows while you are disconnected. For example, taking a few units of basal insulin by injection will help keep glucose levels down during all-day sporting events or days at the beach. You must remember to reconnect and take supplemental insulin because these few units won't replace your full basal dose. You should also make sure that you reduce your total basal rate to compensate for the insulin you already have in your system from the injected insulin.

- **Total pump vacation.** If you want to completely remove your pump, you're going to have to return to MDI therapy. Talk to your health care team before you go back to MDI. To determine your dose of basal insulin by injection, you might want to take your total basal insulin used in the pump and increase it by 10–20%. Your boluses, which you will take by syringe, will be the same as what you took with your pump. If there are different rates used during different time periods, don't forget to follow those patterns. Be very careful not to stack insulin now that you don't have your bolus calculator (which uses active insulin to adjust correction boluses).

- **Emergency discontinuation of insulin pump therapy.** If your pump stops working and it will take a day or two to get a replacement pump, you can manage your diabetes with MDI (go back to basal insulin once or twice a day and boluses for meals and correction) or with rapid-acting insulin only. If you choose to use rapid-acting insulin only, calculate and take your meal and correction boluses the same way you would if you were still on your pump. For your basal rate, you can calculate your basal insulin every two or three hours and take it as an injection at those time intervals.

For example, if you had a basal rate of 1.1 units per hour from 6:00–9:00 A.M., you would take 3.3 units.

If you decide to take a break from the pump (regardless of which replacement method you're using), be very sure that you always have insulin in your system. Insufficient insulin levels can lead to hyperglycemia and the development of ketones. Talk to your health care team if you want to take an extended vacation from the pump or if you decide the pump is not for you. They will help you return to the best diabetes management therapy for you.

PUMP DISCONNECTION GUIDELINES

1. Monitor glucose every two hours.

2. Consider taking a bolus equal to the basal insulin being missed (calculated as your basal rate multiplied by the number of hours you are off the pump) every two to three hours.

3. Reconnect for meals and corrections OR take insulin by syringe.

CHAPTER REVIEW

➡ Sick-day management is critical when you are on an insulin pump. Be sure you have a protocol to follow and all the supplies you need, including a way to check ketones in blood or in urine. Start a log sheet, check glucose often (every 30–60 minutes initially), stay hydrated (drinking fluids matters more than eating), check ketones, check pump site and tubing, and be sure you have help. Contact your diabetes team as soon as is needed.

➡ If you have unexplained high or low glucose levels, go into troubleshooting mode. Check infusion sites, the tubing, the reservoir, the insulin (it may have expired or been exposed to excessive heat or cold), your pump settings, your recent insulin delivery history, and whether the pump is properly functioning.

➡ It is important for someone using insulin pump therapy to understand that he or she can develop ketones if the pump stops delivering insulin. Because you no longer have long-acting or basal insulin in your body, ketones may form as soon as three hours after the insulin infusion is interrupted. You develop ketones when you do not have enough insulin in the bloodstream—even if you have been taking your usual doses but it doesn't meet your metabolic needs. This occurs with infection, stress, or illness. Most frequently, hyperglycemia and ketones go hand in hand, but you may have only mild hyperglycemia, a normal glucose level, or even a low glucose level and still have ketones.

➡ You need to work with your diabetes team and other health care providers to know what to do with your insulin pump if you are hospitalized.

➡ If your pump stops working, it might take a day or two to get a replacement pump. You can manage your diabetes with rapid-acting insulin only. Calculate your meal and correction boluses the same way you would if you were still on your pump. For your basal rate, you will need to calculate how much insulin you need to take every two to three hours to replace your basal rate and then determine how much to give as injections. You might want to replace your basal insulin with a shot of long-acting insulin every 12 or 24 hours.

CHAPTER 10

TRAVEL WITH THE PUMP

Traveling with diabetes requires planning, and traveling with the pump requires even a bit more planning. The good news is that the pump allows for easier adjustments and will likely give you better diabetes control while you travel. You can adjust your basal rates, alter your boluses, and adjust the clock on the pump. You can adjust your insulin administration if you are increasing or decreasing your activity levels during specific parts of the day (e.g., walking around a big city, hiking or backpacking, or being sedentary on road trips). You can easily give yourself correction boluses for foreign foods or if you're treating yourself to local snacks and desserts (like crepes in France or gelato in Italy). There are a few key things that you must always remember when traveling while on the pump. By arming yourself with knowledge and by being prepared, worldwide travel will be what you always dreamed it would be.

ALWAYS BE PREPARED

Travel requires extra vigilance with diabetes management, no matter what therapy you are on. Crossing time zones, sampling new foods, frequent changes in activity level, and the everyday stress of travel (airport security, rushing to catch a train, or waiting in endless lines) can all affect your glucose levels. The number one rule for safe travel is to check your glucose levels frequently and to always be prepared to treat with extra food or insulin.

When you are on MDI, you must always have adequate amounts of extra insulin and syringes with you when you travel. This is a good idea if you're leaving town even for the day. With the pump, it is a good idea to bring a few more things with you as well. Below is a list of the items that you should always have in a backpack or travel kit for any kind of travel.

- **Pump emergency card.** This is a card given to you by most pump companies. It has your name, your device name and details, and treatment recommendations should something happen to you. This information can also come from your health care team.

- **Extra sets.** Pack two or more, depending on how long you'll be gone. If the set you're using when you leave fails and then for some reason your backup fails too, then you will still have a backup. When you travel for more than a few nights, you might want to think of bringing two sets for every three days of travel. It may seem like a lot, but it's better to be prepared than to be without a set.

  ➡ For every set you bring, you'll also want to bring a reservoir. You might not need quite as many reservoirs because they usually aren't the parts that malfunction.

- **Syringes or insulin pens.** A couple of syringes will be necessary if you are in a situation where you are unable to change a set and your blood glucose levels are inexplicably high. Syringes are also necessary if you develop ketones. You could opt to carry insulin pens with rapid-acting insulin if you'd rather pack those than syringes and vials.

- **Extra vial(s) of rapid-acting insulin.** If you are gone for longer than one to two weeks, you might want to think about taking two vials. This is especially important if you are traveling somewhere abroad and are unable to get your prescriptions filled easily if something goes wrong. Be sure that the insulin has not expired.

- **A vial of basal insulin.** If you are comfortable using long-acting insulins or happen to have some on hand, bring them with you while traveling in case you need to return to MDI therapy. Your insulin must have a current prescription on the box. This will prove that you have a justifiable reason for carrying all of your other medical equipment and syringes. Be sure that the insulin has not expired.

- **Extra strips.** You will always need extra test strips when traveling. You can't correct or give accurate insulin adjustments without the ability to test.
    - ⇒ If you're going abroad, it's wise to bring another blood glucose meter and batteries. These will be needed if any part of your current kit fails or if you want to leave a kit in your room and have one to take on outings.

- **Extra tape, appropriate fluids or wipes, and other application or removal aids.** Basically, the rule is "If you use it at home, bring it along." If you use a preparation to remove tape adhesive or to protect your sites at home, then you're going to want it when you're traveling. Also, bringing extra tape is a good idea even if you don't normally use it. Vacationing and traveling often throw you into situations where your tubing could get pulled out or your sets could be damaged. That little bit of extra security tape might just save you a dislodged catheter and a high glucose level.

- **Extra batteries.** Make sure you have extra batteries for your pump as well as for your test kit (and your CGM, if you have one). You don't want to go searching for batteries on your vacation. Keeping a few handy will guarantee that you won't be stuck with a pump and no means to power it.

- **A way to safely dispose of sharps.** It might be inconvenient to bring your small sharps container or some other container to safely dispose of your used needles but it is important. Don't forget, safety precautions should be followed everywhere.

- **Ketone testing equipment.** Whether it is foil-wrapped strips, a vial, or a blood ketone monitor, you must have a way to check for ketones when traveling.

- **Glucagon with a prescription.** Transportation Security Administration (TSA) officials may check your bag of supplies. In order to have your glucagon approved for travel, you must show a prescription for it in your name and it must not be expired.

- **Food, glucose tabs, etc.** Be sure to have food, glucose tabs, glucose gel, or whatever you need to treat low glucose levels.

- **Loaner or travel pump.** Some companies will send you an extra insulin pump as a "travel pump" in case something happens to yours while you are away. It can cost around $50, and for some companies must be insured, but this extra pump can be a lifesaver if yours breaks, is misplaced, or is stolen. These pumps are usually only available for international travel because you can get a pump within 24 hours if you are still in the U.S.

AIRPORTS AND INTERNATIONAL TRAVEL

International air travel with medical devices can be difficult if security personnel are not familiar with insulin pumps. Give yourself *plenty of time* before your flight leaves so you don't miss it if you are delayed for security reasons. It is important to have the printed prescription for all of your diabetes supplies with you when you travel. These prescriptions can be taken off insulin boxes, the box for your insulin syringes, and the box for your pump supplies, and placed in a bag or other container. The prescriptions must match your name on your identification, such as your driver's license or passport. A note from the doctor on official stationery might also be helpful. However, because these are so easily forged, it is more important to show that you have prescriptions for all of your medications.

SEPARATE YOUR INSULIN VIALS

Sometimes it is smart to put a vial of insulin in a different location, so if one of them gets lost or is ruined by heat or cold, you still have another good one.

NO X-RAYS FOR YOUR DEVICES

Your pump and CGM should NOT go through the x-ray machine. However, they can pass through the metal detector.

You might also be stopped if you have a CGM device, which has a separate controller. Neither the pump nor the receiver should go through the x-ray machine. This usually means that security staff will need to inspect you by hand. Often they will do a search or swab all of your carry-ons. Rarely, they will do full pat-down inspections. If these occur, they may take extra time.

Talk to your health care team before you plan on leaving the country, because they may be able to tell you how to manage prescriptions or emergencies in other countries. Another helpful contact is your health insurance company. They may be able to assist you in finding places where you can buy supplies or insulin if you need them. Some pump companies make pumps and supplies that have similar names in other countries, but they do not work with U.S. pumps. It may be helpful to know about this before you leave home.

If you are worried about communication problems with security personnel abroad, you might want to translate your doctor's note or other important information into that country's language before you leave.

TRAVELING ACROSS TIME ZONES

If you're traveling across time zones, you will likely experience jetlag. Jetlag not only means difficulty adjusting to a new sleeping pattern; it also means your body has to change its metabolic and hormone secretion patterns that are associated with your sleep/wake cycles. Your liver releases stored glucose at different rates depending on whether you are awake or asleep. Having the ability to adjust your basal rates with the pump can really help with glucose control when you are jetlagged.

If you're taking a short or long trip or anything in between, then you can probably just change your pump time during travel to the time at your destination (for example, if you're going from Los Angeles to New York, a three-hour time change, then you can just change the time on your pump during your flight or once you land).

Your goal should be to establish your sleep/wake cycle to match where you are, and this is the same goal for your basal rate timing as well. Check more often to be sure.

OTHER COMMON TRAVEL ACTIVITIES

It's common to exercise more when you travel. Watch your basal rates and blood glucose levels closely and always bring extra food in case you go low. Glucose tabs are surprisingly difficult to find abroad or even in some places in the U.S., so bringing a good supply with you is a smart idea. Bring enough treatments for hypoglycemia so you can treat yourself until you find something to buy locally. Another good idea is to bring snack bars or some kind of snack that has starch and protein so you always have enough glucose in your blood. These are nice also for "meals" in airports or for times when you're unable to find food and you need to eat.

Camping and Skiing

When camping, you need to consider altitude, temperature, physical activity, and food supply. Be sure you can control the temperatures that the insulin in your pump, your extra insulin vials, and other critical supplies are exposed to. If you are carrying these supplies with you at all times, you might want to think about getting temperature-controlled packs for cooling and protective covering to avoid freezing. A small lunchbox with an ice pack can keep your insulin and supplies at acceptable temperatures for a few days, as long as it is not placed in direct sunlight (this might turn it into a small oven!). In freezing weather, keep your pump, tubing, and supplies inside your coat and next to your body, where they will be kept warm. (This also applies if you live somewhere with harsh winters).

Altitude changes can create air bubbles or increase their frequency, so check your tubing often. Altitude, exercise, and camping food can also affect the amount of insulin you need. Talk to your diabetes team about reducing your basal rates and boluses, when to suspend, and how to adjust your doses as your trip progresses. Don't forget to check your glucose often and in the middle of the night to reduce your risk of severe hypoglycemia.

Beach Days

When you go to the beach, you will need to plan on disconnecting from your pump and consider your activity level and how you will protect your pump and infusion set from heat, sand, and water. Everyone knows that sand gets everywhere and can disrupt your insulin pump and insertion sites. If you remove your pump, think about placing it in a plastic bag in a cooler. This protects it from sand and keeps your insulin from overheating in the sun. Remember, ice packs can freeze insulin if they are in direct contact—this should be avoided. Also be careful not to submerge your pump in water unless you are sure it is waterproof.

Most infusion sets come with clip-on safety covers for the insertion site. These are very handy because sand will creep into the attachment's crevices and prevent a complete connection when you decide to put your pump back on or when you take a correction bolus. You don't have to worry about sand or sea water getting into your body when you're swimming, though, even if you don't have the safety cover. These sets are designed to let in only insulin via the tubing, and the catheter will not let in water, other liquids, or sand. It should also be noted that the safety cover will not prevent a set from being pulled out, so bring an extra couple of sets. As always, check your blood glucose often to be sure you won't spoil a great beach day with fluctuating glucose levels.

Amusement Parks

A day at the amusement park can be harder to manage than you might think. You need to consider the temperature, your activity level, hydration, food choices, and a whole lot of adrenaline. Waiting in long lines in the sun can lead to overheating—of you, your pump, and your insulin. See if the park has a program for people with special needs; this might help reduce the time you spend waiting in lines. Watch your food choices, drink plenty of water, check your glucose levels often (particularly after you have been screaming on rides that turn you upside down and have you going at extraordinary speeds). Under these conditions, anything can happen to your glucose levels, so be cautious. Don't overcorrect those highs from an adrenaline rush. They usually don't last very long.

Are We There Yet? Long Trips by Car, Plane, Boat, or Train

When you are traveling a long distance over a long time period, consider what happens when you get almost no exercise. During long trips, you get less exercise than usual, even if you have a desk job. You hardly move your muscles. In turn, your muscles don't use much glucose, possibly causing your insulin requirements to increase. For long road trips, you might need to increase your basal rates or take more insulin for your correction and food boluses. This is a good time to consider a temporary increase in basal rates, by 10–20% initially (110–120% basal rate), and then increase as needed depending on your glucose levels.

Watch your food choices for your snacks and meals. We all know that road trips, train stations, and airports are filled with less-than-healthy food choices. Combined with lack of activity, these foods might increase your glucose to a higher number faster than usual. Test often, bolus before you eat, and drink plenty of fluids to help manage your glucose levels during your travels.

CHAPTER REVIEW

➡ Travel requires extra vigilance. Crossing time zones, eating new foods, changing activity levels, and the everyday stresses of travel can all affect your glucose levels. The first rule for safe travel is to check your glucose levels frequently and to be prepared at all times to treat with extra food or insulin.

➡ Getting through the airport can be difficult. Be prepared for delays at security and know that you pump and CGM should NOT go through the x-ray machine. But they can pass through the metal detector.

➡ Crossing time zones can be difficult for anyone. Your goal should be to establish your sleep/wake pattern to match where you are, and this is the same goal for your basal rate timing as well.

➡ Doing everything everyone else does should be your goal. Being prepared—having sufficient supplies, checking glucose levels often, and factoring in your activity level—will help you have safe diabetes management wherever you go.

CHAPTER 11

THE PUMP AT SCHOOL
FROM THE BEGINNING THROUGH COLLEGE

Diabetes must be managed 24 hours a day, seven days a week. This means that diabetes must be effectively managed at school too. Because careful monitoring of glucose levels must occur throughout the school day and insulin must be administered, it is important to have coordination and collaboration between the students, parents, school nurses, teachers, school administrators, and the diabetes health care team. This is best accomplished through meetings, familiarity with regulations, and a written diabetes management plan, regardless of whether the student uses an insulin pump or injection therapy. In this way, the student with diabetes can be safe, have optimal diabetes management, and be able to have a positive and rewarding school experience.

School personnel—most importantly the school nurse and teachers—must understand the basics of diabetes as well as of insulin pump therapy. You need to understand your rights under the Americans with Disabilities Act. Together you must devise the plan that allows for you or your child to be effectively and safely managed in school.

There are valuable resources available. Visit the Safe at School page on the American Diabetes Association's website (www.diabetes.org/safeatschool). Be sure to also read *Helping the Student with Diabetes Succeed: A Guide for School Personnel*, which is available on the National Diabetes Education Program website (www.ndep.nih. gov/media/youth_ndepschoolguide.pdf).

YOUR PERSONAL DIABETES MEDICAL MANAGEMENT PLAN

There are three management plans that you must devise for the school. They outline exactly what is required for success with diabetes and insulin pump therapy.

1. **Diabetes Medical Management Plan (DMMP).** The DMMP is completed by the student's diabetes health care team and contains the medical orders that are the basis for the student's health care and education plans.

2. **Individualized Health Plan (IHP).** This plan is developed by the school nurse in collaboration with the student's diabetes health care team and family to put the medical recommendations in the student's DMMP into practice in the school.

3. **Emergency care plans for hypoglycemia and hyperglycemia.** These emergency care plans are based on the medical orders, summarize how to recognize and treat hypoglycemia and hyperglycemia, and describe whom to contact for help. These plans, developed by the school nurse, should be distributed to all school personnel who are responsible for the student with diabetes during the school day and during school-sponsored activities.

The DMMP is set up between your diabetes care team, the school nurse, and you (and your child). The school will require a written assessment of the child's diabetes health. It will cover all of the actions required for blood glucose testing, treating hypoglycemia and hyperglycemia, eating, exercising, ketone testing, field trips, delivery of boluses, pump disconnections, who is to treat the student in emergencies, and any other necessary medical information about managing glucose levels (this includes the child's ability to treat himself or herself independently, other medications, mental conditions, and hypoglycemia unawareness). The DMMP must be absolutely accurate, updated often, and always available because the nurse will use this to determine the Individualized Health Plan's (IHP) strategies for diabetes care at school and a 504 Plan or Individualized Education Plan (IEP), if used (covered in Federal Laws, later in this chapter).

Members of the School Health Team	Members of the Student's Diabetes Health Care Team
Student with diabetes	Student with diabetes
Parent(s)/guardian	Parent(s)/guardian
School nurse	Doctor
Other school health care personnel	Nurse
Trained diabetes personnel	Registered dietitian
Administrators	Diabetes educator
Principal	Other health care providers involved with
504 Plan/Individualized Education Plan	the student's diabetes care
(IEP) coordinator	
Office staff	
Student's teacher(s)	
Guidance counselor	
Coach, lunchroom and other school staff	

A DMMP should include details about the child's overall diabetes care and pump use. It is a guideline and is meant to provide instructions for common concerns or issues that are related to diabetes. There is no way to predict everything that might happen, and the DMMP should not be viewed as a complete, inflexible instruction manual. Parents or guardians can override the DMMP if they need to, and they should always be contacted if there are any questions or concerns about a child's treatment.

Here is a list of information that should always be included in the DMMP. Sample forms for a DMMP are available on the websites noted in this section.

→ **Child's information.** Include child's name, date of birth, classroom/grade, address, home phone, parent/guardian's cell or work phone.

→ **Current diabetes information.** Include date of diagnosis, current A1C, level of diabetes awareness (a younger child's ability to recognize high or low blood glucose, an older child's independent abilities, knowledge of the pump's capabilities, etc.), overall diabetes health, types of insulins used, and the brand, serial number, and model names for the blood glucose meter, insulin pump, and

CGM (if used). The phone number for the help line for the pump and CGM device (if used) should also be included.

➡ **Diabetes doctor's contact information.** Include doctor's name, phone number, and location of practice. Include this information for other health care providers, such as nurses, physician assistants, and nurse practitioners.

➡ **Emergency contact information.** This might include you or another guardian, a separate family member, or a friend who can also assist in the case of an emergency if you cannot be reached.

➡ **Specific instructions.** These instructions will change depending on the child's age and capabilities with his or her own diabetes care. This section should be updated very often and will include:

- **Assistance with blood glucose monitoring and logging.** How to do it, where to record it, and when and where it takes place.

- **Instructions for hypoglycemia.** Definition of and treatment for mild, moderate, and severe lows. When and how to disconnect the pump.

- **Instructions for hyperglycemia.** List the child's ISF, describe whether insulin is to be given by pump or syringe, detail ketone testing, and indicate when infusion sets should be changed.

- **How and when to administer glucagon.**

- **How and when to check for ketones.**

- **Instructions for meal and snack boluses.** List the child's ICRs. Define who counts the carbs, who enters them into the pump, and who approves giving insulin. Also note whether a dual-wave or square-wave bolus should be used for specific foods and how that is done.

- **Pump storage.**

- **Temporary basals for physical activity (if needed).**

- **CGM care and usage.** Describe when a calibration is needed and how to do it.

- **How to change an infusion set.** Describe how to fill the reservoir, prime the tubing, and connect and fill the cannula.

➡ **All medications kept and administered at school.** This includes insulin and any other medications, for diabetes or other conditions.

➡ **Typical symptoms.** This should cover both hypoglycemia and hyperglycemia and should also include whether the child is able to recognize those symptoms.

➡ **List of supplies and equipment worn and used daily.** This might also include a list of what the child should keep at school as well as which supplies are kept in each room/area (e.g., supplies for changing sets and insulin in the nurse's office, blood glucose test kit and treatment for hypoglycemia in the classroom, and treatment for hypoglycemia in a gym locker or with the gym teacher).

➡ **Special field trips and excursion instructions.**

➡ **Sharps and sharps disposal.**

➡ **Other medical information.** Include allergies, other conditions (such as celiac disease), mental diagnosis, and psychological diagnosis.

Federal Laws

You should familiarize yourself with the three federal laws that address the school's responsibilities to help students with diabetes:

MANAGING YOUR DMMP

An updated copy of the DMMP should be kept with the school nurse, homeroom teacher, and parents at all times. In the beginning of every year, the DMMP should be revised, reviewed, and signed by all necessary individuals (this might include a diabetes educator, a school administrator, the guardians, a school nurse, and the homeroom teacher).

Section 504 of the Rehabilitation Act of 1973 (Section 504), the Americans with Disabilities Act of 1990 (ADA), and the Individuals with Disabilities Education Act (IDEA). These federal laws provide a framework for planning and implementing effective diabetes management in the school setting, for preparing the student's education plan, and for protecting the student's privacy. The requirements of federal laws must always be met. School administrators and nursing personnel also should determine whether applicable state and local laws need to be factored into helping students with diabetes.

The school will work with you to meet the federal regulations. Your child should develop a 504 Plan or an IEP to ensure that his or her medical and academic needs will be met. The 504 Plan sets out an agreement to make sure the student with diabetes has the same access to education as other children. Students who qualify for services under IDEA will have an IEP instead of a 504 Plan. Typically, an IEP is more specific and focused than a 504 Plan, detailing the student's academic needs, current level of functioning, supports, and goals.

THE PUMP IN THE CLASSROOM

You must determine where you or your child will do glucose monitoring. It is best—if you and your child agree—to check blood glucose levels and treat them within the classroom, anytime and anywhere. Leaving the classroom to go to the nurse's office or elsewhere means that the child may be without supervision while going to check, that there could be a delay in finding and treating high and low glucose levels, and that classroom time and instruction will be missed. You also need to consider where you want bolus insulin administration to occur: in the classroom, the lunchroom, or someplace else, such as the nurse's office. Finally, you need to consider where you want infusion set changes to occur and other medications given, likely not in the classroom. Allowing diabetes tasks (particularly with the pump) to occur anytime and anyplace helps normalize these procedures as well as improve the skills of the child.

INDEPENDENCE AND CONFIDENCE

The ability to test and treat in the classroom, lunchroom, gymnasium, and elsewhere makes checking blood glucose (either by blood or sensor) a normal part of the school day. When a child is allowed to test in the classroom, the child with diabetes as well as his or her peers will view testing as a regular activity.

Teachers, substitutes, and other school personnel (principals, counselors, etc.) should be aware that the pump is not a pager, MP3 player, or game. The child might also need access to a cell phone to discuss management issues with a parent.

Security When Disconnecting

During class, if the student needs to disconnect the pump for a time, there needs to be a designated area to safely store the pump that is in a cool, dry place and that can be secured so that the pump cannot be taken or tampered with. For gym class, if the DMMP designates disconnecting the pump, a locker that can be secured, the gym teacher's office, or the nurse's office are good choices for safe storage. Unfortunately, pumps, glucose meters, and other diabetes equipment can be stolen.

Field Trips

No child should be prohibited from a school activity because of diabetes. However, special considerations need to be in place to ensure that there is adequate supervision for diabetes management and the pump.

Meal and Snack Time

It is the obligation of the school to provide nutrition information for the foods offered. With appropriate nutrition information, the child (if he or she is capable) or the responsible adult in the school can ensure that the correct amount of insulin is taken. Other foods such as snacks and treats that are not part of the school's official meal policies should have nutrition information made available if possible.

School Schedule

The school schedule, with regard to meals, snacks, gym class, and recess, should be discussed by the parents and school personnel. Adjustments in the diabetes regimen—and the school schedule, if needed—should be made to help the child successfully manage blood glucose levels.

Extra Supplies

Extra supplies should always be kept at school. There should be enough to last 72 hours, in case there is a natural disaster or an emergency that lasts a few days. Supplies should be stored in a secure area but should also be easily accessible. Most often, they are kept in the nurse's office. If a child needs to use an infusion set or other supplies from the supply cache, be aware that they need to be replaced to remain properly stocked. Check in with the nurse every few weeks to make sure that there is always the proper amount of supplies. Supplies should include

- insulin (rapid- and perhaps long-acting)
- syringes and/or pen needles
- infusion sets
- reservoirs
- tape
- adhesive aids and/or removing agents
- extra blood glucose monitor and lancet
- extra test strips
- extra lancets
- batteries for the pump, blood glucose meter, and cgm
- any insertion device needed for infusion sets or syringes
- urine ketone strips or blood ketone monitor
- fast-acting carbohydrates (such as juice, glucose tabs, or glucose gel) and snacks with protein (such as peanut butter or cheese crackers, granola bars) for treating lows
- glucagon
- emergency contact information, doctor's information.

Discussing the Pump at School

For elementary school children, diabetes and the insulin pump can awaken curiosity. Friends and classmates often want to ask many questions, touch the pump, and figure out what it does. As long as it is okay with the child, arrange a "show-and-tell" about diabetes and the pump. It is important, however, to make sure that your child feels safe and comfortable with the idea of a presentation because many children are shy about their diabetes. If a show-and-tell introduction to the class is embarrassing for your child, discuss how he or she would like to deal with curious classmates. One option is to write a letter that goes home with classmates. By preparing the child for these types of scenarios, you may be able to teach them more about diabetes, and they might acquire a sense of pride when they can explain what diabetes is and how the pump helps them live a normal life.

Special Accommodations

During school examinations, your child will still need access to testing equipment, a source of glucose, and insulin via the pump. Accommodations for this should be discussed before examinations begin. The student might be placed in a separate room and should be allowed to manage his or her diabetes without that influencing the exam results. For timed examinations, the time needed to check glucose levels and possibly correct them should not be counted.

Further Resources

- The American Diabetes Association's webpage covering discrimination at school and work has several helpful articles on the topic (www.diabetes.org/living-with-diabetes/parents-and-kids/diabetes-care-at-school/position-statements-and-resources-for-care-at-school.html).

- The National Diabetes Education Program has a book that provides sample DMMPs and other forms for schools, parents, and students. It is called *Helping the Student with Diabetes Succeed:*

A Guide for School Personnel and is available at www.ndep.nih. gov/media/youth_ndepschoolguide.pdf.

• Contact the pump company if you have questions about integrating the pump into the school environment. They have a 24-hour help lines that may be a good resource when putting together presentations for classmates, school personnel, or teachers. Pump manufacturers can also provide specific pump information for the DMMP.

COLLEGE WITH AN INSULIN PUMP

Having an insulin pump during college can help manage the ups and downs, crazy schedules, fast food, stress, and all the other things that college life offers. Insulin pump therapy allows you to be flexible with your diabetes care while still maintaining good control. If you know how to use your pump's key features and have good knowledge of how your body reacts to different treatments, then you have the resources to succeed with the pump during school.

Even without diabetes, college is a turbulent time that will force you to adapt and roll with the punches. Sports, classes, tests, homework, on-campus dining (and off-campus dining, for that matter), dorm life, new places, and new people will all affect blood glucose and diabetes care. It can be tricky, but with a little practice the pump will allow you to sail through with good blood glucose levels (and good grades as well).

The Schedule that Isn't One

For many students in college, their schedule varies from day to day. Some days require getting up much earlier than others, and some days require sitting in several classes back-to-back with no breaks for meals. It is a good idea to check basal rates before attending college in order to determine if they are appropriate. After getting your class schedule, think about how to prepare for different days. Maybe three of the five days include a sport; you might want to make a new basal pattern for those days. Do you have four back-to-back classes that prohibit lunch? For those days, making sure you have adequate snacks is important, or you should pack a lunch to eat on the go. Unexpected schedule disruptions like long study sessions often include lots of snacking, which can increase your blood glucose. Make sure you administer sufficient insulin to cover these snacks. Stress may also play a role in your diabetes management.

Alcohol

Alcohol can be found on any college campus—despite the fact that underage drinking is illegal. Alcohol affects glucose levels and can lead to severe hypoglycemia.

When alcohol is ingested, it decreases the ability of the liver to release stored glucose. If a large amount of alcohol is ingested without food, particularly before bedtime, there is the risk of severe hypoglycemia during sleep and even the next day. Therefore, if you decide to drink, plan on reducing insulin doses, eating, checking glucose often, and being sure someone around you knows that you have diabetes. The best plan, however, is never to drink in excess.

Your Dorm, Your Resident Assistant, and Your Roommate

Having a roommate or roommates is part of college life. When you're getting to know each other, you should tell your roommate about your diabetes. At a minimum, he or she needs to know about hypoglycemia, what you will look and act like, and what they can to do help (if you want them to) or to call 911 if you are unresponsive or confused.

In addition, tell them about the pump. Explain what it does and that you will almost always be wearing it. Answer any questions they might have. If you share a refrigerator, let them know that your insulin is what keeps you alive and that it is not to be tampered with; the same goes for your supplies for glucose monitoring and for the pump. Also assure them that you will follow the universal safety precautions for your sharps from the infusion set, lancets, and syringes. The more you can tell them, the safer your living situation will be. You must also tell the resident assistant in your dorm that you have diabetes and inform him or her of what should be done in an emergency. Of course, you should consider sharing the fact that you have diabetes with new friends as well.

Health Services

You should go to health services when you arrive on campus. Let them know that you have diabetes and that you use an insulin pump. Give them information about your diabetes history, your present insulin doses, and your overall management plan. Give them the names and numbers of your diabetes team and make them a part of the network of your diabetes care providers.

Running Out of Supplies

For some, going to college means that they will be in charge of their supplies for the first time. Parents can't always check in to remind you about reordering your supplies. Discussing how to refill prescriptions for pump supplies, insulin, and test strips is vital. Sit down and brainstorm ways to remember to reorder your supplies. If you are left with only one or two infusion sets, you will not have enough time to refill your order by mail. Try imposing the "last box" rule. This means that whenever you notice you are about to open your last box of supplies, you order more—right away. If you are a procrastinator, use the "second-to-last-box" rule. Do a test run of ordering supplies before leaving for college so you are comfortable with this routine.

CHAPTER REVIEW

➡ A DMMP should include details about the child's overall diabetes care and pump use. It is a guideline and is meant to serve as instructions for common concerns or issues related to diabetes at school.

➡ The ability to test and treat in the classroom, lunchroom, gymnasium, and other places makes checking blood glucose (either by blood or sensor) and diabetes management a normal part of the school day. The child with diabetes as well as his or her peers will view managing diabetes as a regular activity.

➡ Having an insulin pump during college can help manage the ups and downs, crazy schedules, fast food, stress, and all the other things that college life offers.

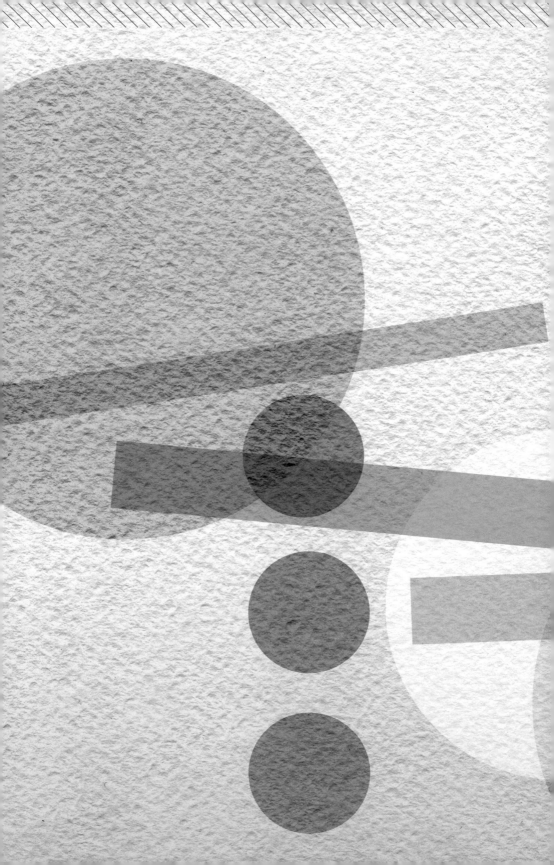

ADJUSTING TO INSULIN PUMP THERAPY

CHAPTER 12

CAPABILITIES BY AGE

Depending on your age (or your child's age), some tasks for diabetes management and pump therapy will require assistance. The assistance can be in the form of either technical or cognitive assistance. But remember, it is always important that someone stays involved, is aware of how diabetes control is progressing, and is there to offer help (e.g., to ask about glucose control and overall psychological adjustment). Diabetes is just too big—even for the most capable adult—to deal with alone.

DEVELOPMENT AND COGNITIVE SKILLS BY AGE RANGE

Helping your child develop the skills and confidence necessary to assume age-appropriate responsibility for his or her own pump and diabetes management requires both of you to work together on this important goal. In some instances, parents may be reluctant to give more responsibility to their children, and some children may be hesitant to take it. Other parents may be anxious to turn over responsibility, sometimes even when the child is not ready to assume it. The goal is to encourage, support, and facilitate your child doing what he or she is able to and what should be done with managing diabetes and the pump.

Children of all ages can begin to participate in their own care according to their abilities and developmental capabilities. Doing this will lead to the ultimate goal of enabling the young adult to leave home—when the time comes—able to manage his or her diabetes safely and effectively. By offering your encouragement and help all along the way, expecting your child to do what is appropriate for their age, and supporting them in doing it, you will prepare your child for their eventual autonomy.

SPECIAL ISSUES FOR ADOLESCENTS AND YOUNG ADULTS

It can be particularly hard for adolescents and young adults to adjust to the rigors of the diabetes regimen. This is because they don't want to be different. They want to lead a "normal" life, and they want to start taking care of themselves more and more. Although diabetes cannot stand in the way of increasing independence and autonomy, diabetes cannot be ignored either. Having an insulin pump may make it easier or harder, depending on what the issues are for the individual and his or her family. There are many things to consider, ranging from physiological (physical functions) to psychological (mental functions). Teens and young adults need encouragement, supervision, and even involvement in their lives and diabetes care.

Physiological

The changes in hormone levels and rapid physical growth that occur during puberty increase insulin resistance. When coupled with an increase in calorie intake, which is normal to meet the physical demands of growth, children in puberty may need to significantly increase their insulin dosages, adjust for the dawn phenomenon, and increase the number of times they bolus each day. Menstruation may result in changes in insulin dosages too. Some girls see high glucose levels before they get their period every month, and they often aren't aware of the reason. Having an insulin pump can make these adjustments easier.

Diabetes Skills and Knowledge by Developmental Age

Age	Skills	Knowledge
Birth to 3 years	• Rapid changes in cognitive and motor skills, nutrition requirements, sleep/wake patterns, and acquisition of developmental milestones	• Inherent trust in parents/caregivers
3–5 years	• Lack motor skills and cognitive ability	• Minimal understanding of diabetes procedures and management issues • Start to ask about food
6–9 years	• Help insert pump catheter • Wear pump appropriately • Protect the catheter site • Unhook pump to give to supervising adult • Reconnect pump, with assistance • Activate bolus dose, with direction	• Understand glucose numbers • Understand importance of blood glucose control • Minimally explain diabetes • Ask about food • May feel different from peers
10–12 years	• Protect pump during activity • Be responsible for pump when unhooked • Insert pump catheter • Hook and unhook pump • Activate bolus dose	• Count carbs • Start to calculate insulin dose for meals and corrections using bolus calculator • Understand that exercise leads to lows
13–14 years	• Suspend basal dose • Program basal rates, with assistance	• Calculate and deliver bolus • Understand the role of exercise • Recognize if basal rates need to be adjusted
15–18 years	• Program changes in basal rates	• Determine what factors affect basal rates and how to check • Determine what new basal rates should be given, with assistance • Determine what factors affect bolus doses • Change algorithm for bolus doses, with assistance • Use sick-day protocol, with assistance

Psychological

The psychological issues that arise during adolescence are often centered on issues of independence. Driving, staying out late, sleeping over at friends' houses, going off to summer programs and camps and eventually college, make it imperative that the adolescent and family are in agreement on how they will meet these new challenges. It is also critical that diabetes doesn't become an excuse to hold the teen back from what are the normal processes of increasing independence. It is equally important that the teen realize that he or she has to effectively manage diabetes if he or she is to gain and deserve more independence and autonomy.

Driving

Being able to drive is a great milestone and achievement. But driving is also dangerous and can be more dangerous if glucose levels aren't managed. Driving is a privilege that must be earned by gaining experience behind the wheel, learning the rules, and passing a test. For someone with diabetes, it must be earned by showing that glucose control and monitoring are done consistently and reliably before getting behind the wheel.

Alcohol

Drinking alcohol is different for people with diabetes. Alcohol can have a profound effect on blood glucose levels and must only be consumed by adults (it is illegal for underage teens to drink). However, even though it is illegal, many teens (even younger ones) drink alcohol, and some do it more than just rarely.

Alcohol can lead to both hyperglycemia and hypoglycemia. Certain alcoholic drinks contain a lot of carbohydrate because they are mixed with fruit juices or sugary sodas or because they contain carbohydrate themselves (beers and sweet wines). Mixers can elevate blood glucose soon after drinking. It is best to avoid covering for these carbohydrates because alcohol has a tendency to cause hypoglycemia later. Alcohol reduces glucose release from the liver and can lead to hypoglycemia between meals and overnight. To compensate, you should eat a snack or meal when you drink and not take insulin for the carbohydrates or at least reduce your insulin dose significantly. Increased monitoring, waking up in the middle of the night to check your glucose and health status, and telling friends about the effects of alcohol can help make it safe to drink in moderation (if you are of legal age).

CHAPTER REVIEW

➡ The tasks required for insulin pump therapy increase as a child ages and gains experience with diabetes. Some parents find it hard to give up any responsibility for diabetes care, whereas others can't wait to give their child more responsibility, sometimes when the child is not ready or able. Issue new responsibilities based on your child's development and abilities. By offering your encouragement and help, as well as considering what diabetes tasks your child is prepared for and ready to take on, you can help ensure a safe transition to adulthood.

➡ Teens need supervision, encouragement, and parental involvement in their lives, as well as in their diabetes management.

CHAPTER 13

ATTITUDES ABOUT THE PUMP

Adapting to life with the insulin pump can be difficult and have an effect on your day-to-day mood and ability to succeed with insulin pump therapy. Learning all that you can about the mechanics of the pump is different from psychologically dealing with the pump. Adjusting to it can be difficult and take time, but when you balance the positives and negatives, the positives hopefully will come out on top.

One major issue for every pump wearer to decide is who should know about the insulin pump and when and how to show or tell them about it. The scenarios for family, friends, and strangers are different. Here are some things to think about when considering the reluctance or hesitancy you may feel about sharing that you wear a pump.

OVERALL ATTITUDES

Having diabetes, adjusting to a chronic illness with a complex treatment regimen, and experiencing hypoglycemia and hyperglycemia can be difficult. People go through several emotions—denial, anger, and depression—especially with first diagnosed. For some people, these emotions come back over and over again. Starting on an insulin pump can bring back these emotions. There is a physical thing attached to the body that serves as a constant reminder that you have diabetes. If you have these emotions, it is important to talk to your diabetes team. Discuss your feelings with them and see if you need to talk to a psychologist, psychiatrist, or social worker. Talk to your parents, other family members, and friends too. This can help, even

> **DETECT DEPRESSION**
>
> If your feelings are affecting your day-to-day living, then you need to discuss this with your diabetes team. People with diabetes have higher rates of depression. Get help. It can make a world of difference!

though they might not know what it feels like to have diabetes. They can still listen and offer support.

In addition, try to find a way to talk to others who are like you, with diabetes and a pump. Find a support group, go to a diabetes event, read blogs, search for others at your college, or go to a diabetes camp (as a camper or counselor). This might help you feel like you are not alone.

Approach pump therapy with an open mind. Be sure it is right for you. Work with your family and your health care team. Establish good habits. Make this new part of your journey the best, and then step back and see how much you have learned and hopefully how much better your diabetes management has become.

HOW TO TELL OTHERS

Friends and Family

One of the first things you'll have to decide is how the people who are close to you, such as friends and family, will play a role in your pump therapy. If you live with a friend, spouse, parent, or significant other, encourage him or her to come to pump training sessions and learn about the pump. This will be helpful if you become ill or have an emergency.

You also need to decide how you want the people with whom you live and interact to assist you with your diabetes and your pump. Do you want them to help you remember to bolus before meals, to test often, or to change your infusion set? Or would you prefer that they just know what to do in an emergency? Diabetes is a hard disease to live with if you don't have support, so don't be afraid to ask for help. Everyone needs it!

Your friends and family may be nervous about your pump at the beginning. Giving them a quick demonstration or information about the pump might make them feel more confident. You need to discuss what you want help with and how to handle an emergency.

Acquaintances and Strangers

If you prefer to conceal your pump from acquaintances and strangers, then you should be able to do that. But know that people may ask what the pump is, so it might be a good idea to have a response ready. People may mistake it for something else, like a cell phone. At functions where cell phones or cameras are prohibited, you may be asked to turn it off or leave it outside. A brief explanation is usually all that is needed. Something like: "This it is not a cell phone/camera, but actually an insulin pump for my diabetes. It's a lifesaving medical device that I need to keep on me at all times to avoid becoming very ill."

WEIGHING IT ALL IN THE BALANCE

Balance is the key when dealing with the ups and downs of insulin pump therapy. Often the short-term or immediate issues that develop with the pump can overshadow the positive and often long-term advantages gained. It can be hard to be upbeat and positive about the pump when you're getting used to a new way of life. But don't forget the advantages: better blood glucose numbers, more flexibility, the bolus calculator, and hopefully very few or no shots!

Negatives

The biggest issues include having something attached to your body, trouble concealing the pump, having to troubleshoot if problems de-

NEED HELP? GOT QUESTIONS?

Call your doctor, nurse, diabetes educator, or the pump company. They all want to help you succeed with your insulin pump!

Advantages and Disadvantages of Pump Therapy

Advantages	Disadvantages
Adjustable basal insulin rates	Attached to a machine
These can be set for different times of the day and night.	*Placement on your body might be difficult. Have to deal with tape adhesive.*
Easier to take multiple boluses each day	A constant reminder of diabetes
Bolus calculator	Might be visible in public
Helps make difficult calculations.	*Promotes unwanted questions.*
Able to deliver fractions of a unit of insulin	Remembering to bolus
Improved glucose levels and reduced A1C	Infusion set failures
Fewer injections/needles	*Need to troubleshoot highs.*
Lifestyle flexibility	Machines can fail and break
You have the tools you need on your body	Higher risk for ketones
Easier to be mobile.	Expense of pump
Decreased hypoglycemia	
Less insulin might be needed.	

velop, and forgetting to bolus. Some people are concerned about concealing the pump as well as the constant hassle of finding a place to put it, especially if they prefer not to reveal that they have diabetes and/or an insulin pump. When the pump becomes more of a hassle than an aid, it's nice to know that it's not permanent and that you can take it off if you have a proper alternative insulin therapy.

Another thing that people tend to have issues with is remembering to bolus. This can mean that they forget about it or that they take their bolus late. Teens and adolescents transitioning to managing their own therapy often have a hard time remembering to bolus on time. Excuses (for anyone, not just teens) often include being too busy, not knowing the carb count, not wanting to bolus in front of friends or peers, or simply forgetting.

It is hard getting into the habit of taking a bolus every time you eat, but it's very important. We also know that taking insulin 15–30 minutes before eating is very effective for reducing after-meal highs and that the insulin pump makes bolusing easy to do. But it is hard to remember all the time. You may have to ease into bolusing before eating by starting with one meal (breakfast is usually the easiest; wake up, test, and bolus for your food and blood glucose right away, and then get ready and eat breakfast last). It's important that you develop these good habits and stick to them for the best control.

Sometimes people on the pump get too confident or lax about their habits, which may have been very good at one point. They stop counting carbs and just estimate, or they continually forget to bolus or bolus late or they just stop using the bolus calculator. These habits add up, and over time can really affect your A1C and overall health. The loss of good habits might also lead people to dislike their pump.

Positives

There are obviously positive aspects about an insulin pump, or people wouldn't choose to use them and doctors wouldn't recommend them. These aspects include (and are not limited to) better overall control of blood glucose levels and A1C, flexibility of your schedule, fewer shots, and better safety when it comes to hypoglycemia. All of these things help your overall health, and pumps can enhance or restore vitality to your life.

CHAPTER REVIEW

➡ Adjusting to diabetes and insulin pump therapy can be challenging. Denial, anger, and depression can recur when you begin insulin pump therapy, reminiscent of how you might have felt when you were first diagnosed with diabetes. Involve others and, if need be, get help from a mental health professional.

➡ Talk to others and involve them in understanding your issues with diabetes and with your insulin pump.

➡ When you think of the negatives, remember all of the positives of insulin pump therapy. Negatives can include always being attached to a machine as a constant reminder of diabetes, it can make your diabetes more visible, you can be at a higher risk of ketones if something malfunctions, and pumps are expensive. Positives include: better fine-tuning and control, improved A1C and ultimately overall health, it greatly reduces the number of shots you must take, it decreases the likelihood of hypoglycemia, and insulin pumps can increase your schedule's flexibility.

CONTINUOUS GLUCOSE MONITORING

CHAPTER 14

THE FACTS ABOUT CONTINUOUS GLUCOSE MONITORING

HOW A CGM WORKS AND ITS COMPONENTS

Starting to use a continuous glucose monitor (CGM) is similar to starting on an insulin pump. It takes knowledge, training, motivation, and support from others. A CGM provides a lot of additional information about your blood glucose levels. It checks your glucose numerous times per day, and signals an alert if your levels are outside your target range or if they are increasing or decreasing too fast. A CGM can generate trend graphs of your data, which can be uploaded into computer programs for later analysis. A CGM provides a lot of information, but for it to be helpful, you need to know what to do with the information and how to turn it into action to improve your diabetes outcomes. And of course, this involves your diabetes team.

A CGM measures your glucose level every one to five minutes (depending on the device) all day and all night. This produces far more information than normal self-monitoring of blood glucose (SMBG), which is done four, six, eight, or more times a day. However, a CGM measures glucose in your interstitial tissue, rather than in your blood. The interstitial fluid is the fluid area that surrounds your body's cells. Glucose enters the interstitial tissue as it works its way to your cells, where it can be used for energy. Because a CGM measures glucose in the interstitial fluid and not in the blood, values obtained at the same time from SMBG and CGM may not be identical. This is particularly true when the glucose level is rapidly changing, such as right after a meal or during exercise. For this reason, the real-time numbers displayed on a CGM monitor are actually a little delayed behind the reading of blood glucose. Depending on the rate of change in the blood glucose, the CGM values are generally within 20% of the blood glucose value. Therefore, it is still important to test your blood glucose with a fingerstick at least four to six times a day. *Most importantly, the decision to give insulin or treat a low glucose level should be based on an SMBG reading and not on the value on your CGM.*

Basic Components
The three parts of the CGM system are the sensor, the transmitter, and the receiver/monitor. These three components communicate with each other to provide you with the glucose level in your interstitial fluid. You can get information in real time by looking at the monitor and by getting alerts, and you can review your levels by uploading the data from your CGM to a computer program. Each separate part of the system is critically important for its functioning.

The Sensor
The sensor sits under the skin and is very similar in size and shape to an infusion set cannula. The sensor is inserted with the help of a needle (which is removed after insertion) and an inserter. It is made of a flexible fiber-plastic material that reacts to glucose changes and sends the information to the transmitter. Once inserted, the sensor should be unnoticed and painless. Different sensors have different lengths, between 6 and 15 mm (1/4–3/4 inch) and are injected at either a 45° or a 90° angle. Depending on the sensor, glucose readings are taken every one to five minutes while you are wearing it.

When you first insert the sensor, it takes time to get the sensor in contact with enough interstitial fluid for it to start measuring glu-

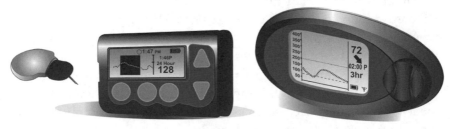

CGM devices.

cose levels. During this "warm-up" time, it does not send glucose values to the transmitter and you will not see any values on the CGM receiver screen. Although it varies depending on which device you use, this warm-up period is generally about two hours.

On the outside, the sensor resembles an infusion set—it has a plastic top covering the sensor and is held to the skin with an adhesive. The transmitter is connected to the plastic part. Sensors generally need to be replaced after three to six or seven days of use, depending on which sensor you use.

The sensor can be placed in a variety of locations on your body, including arms, legs, abdomen, or buttocks. You need enough body fat to be able to accommodate a sensor. A good rule for this is if you can pinch up enough body fat with two fingers to be able to insert a sensor, then that's a good location. If you are someone who does not have many areas with a lot of body fat, you might need to consider the different insertion angles and sensor lengths when choosing a CGM. Another thing to consider is that these are the same areas where infusion sets are worn. There must be at least 2 inches between the infusion set and a sensor. Sensors might not function well in areas that have swollen tissue from repeated insulin administration.

The Transmitter
The transmitter sends information from the sensor to the monitor/ receiver. It clips into the plastic head of the sensor, either on top or on the side, and is generally taped down after connection. Radio-wave or Bluetooth technology sends the readings to the receiver. Depending on the brand, the transmitter can communicate with a receiver that is between 5 and 10 feet away. Sometimes the signal can be blocked or interrupted by cell phones or other transmitting devices, but the signal will be restored automatically once the source of the interruption is removed. Transmitters vary in size (6–12 mm or $1/4$–$1/2$ inch in height) and shape; some are rectangular and some are round.

Transmitters have batteries that need to be replaced or recharged regularly. Most batteries will last through several sensors, and the status of the transmitter battery can be viewed on the receiver. All transmitters are waterproof, so you can shower, bathe, or swim without worrying that they will damaged. If you are swimming, especially in the ocean, you must make sure the transmitters and sensors are securely adhered to your body so you don't lose them.

The Receiver/Monitor

The receiver/monitor is the part of the CGM that displays the current blood glucose level as well as trend arrows, graphs, and device information, such as battery life, transmitter signal strength, date, and time. There are different styles of receivers. Some use the same screen as your insulin pump, so you don't have to carry another device. Handheld receivers can be kept in your pocket, purse, or elsewhere nearby.

CGM systems have alarms to warn you of high and low blood glucose levels. There are alarms that tell you when you need to calibrate your system, and some can tell you when your glucose levels are rising or falling too fast. Alarms will notify you when your battery is running low or when the signal from the transmitter is lost. Like a cell phone, most receivers let you choose between a sound or a vibrating alert. All receivers also have a backlight, so information can be viewed in the dark.

COMMON MISCONCEPTIONS

CGM Replaces SMBG

CGM does not replace SMBG or testing with a glucose meter. This misconception stems from the idea that the CGM monitors blood glucose rather than interstitial glucose levels. In fact, in the beginning, SMBG testing might increase. It is important to perform SMBG at least four to six times per day—even when you wear a CGM—because you have to calibrate the CGM with an SMBG reading and make treatment decisions about insulin doses and hypoglycemia from SMBG readings only.

CGM and Blood Glucose Levels Are Identical

There is a 10- to 20-minute lag between the glucose levels obtained with CGM and those obtained with SMBG. But even with this lag, the CGM values are generally within 20% of the SMBG levels.

Sensors Can Be Worn Infrequently

If you wear the sensor for only a couple of days a month, you may not see the same benefits as someone who wears it continuously. The STAR 3 study (described in chapter 1) showed that when someone wore a CGM for about 60% of the time, A1C was lowered by 0.5%, but when a CGM was worn for 80–100% of the time, there was a 1.2% drop in A1C.

If you don't want to use CGM all of the time, consider using it during illnesses, when glucose management is not optimal, while travelling, or when you change your usual schedule. It may help you better manage your diabetes during these times.

CGM Can Be Kept Private

Using and reviewing the data from a CGM can lead to success, but keeping up with all that data will make it hard to keep your CGM a secret. If you are going to look at the monitor frequently, respond to the alerts, and alter your regimen, people will likely see you using the device. As with the pump, there is no reason to advertise or conceal this important device. If strangers see it, you might want to stop questions by giving an explanation—or have an answer ready if they ask. It is best to have the support of friends and family, because it will make using the CGM and managing your diabetes easier.

CGM Can Be Information Overload

Because CGM gives a lot of information—hundreds of glucose values per day—it takes time to determine how to use the numbers, alerts, and trends to best manage your diabetes. Working with your diabetes team is necessary at the beginning, but as time goes on, you will gain expertise and experience.

No Room on Your Body for Both a CGM and an Insulin Pump

You have enough places on your body for a CGM and an insulin pump. The sensors are about the size of a pump infusion site and must be placed at least 2 inches from a pump site. You rotate the sites like you do with your pump and can use any body area where you can pinch up enough skin with two fingers.

A CGM Must Be Used with a Sensor
Though CGM and pump therapies work very well together, there are many people on multiple daily injection (MDI) therapy who successfully use the CGM to help manage their diabetes.

APPROPRIATE CANDIDATES FOR A CGM

A CGM should be considered if you have wide fluctuations in glucose levels; have frequent, severe, unrecognized, or nocturnal hypoglycemia; have trouble with glucose control during exercise or periods of stress; have not achieved your target A1C; or want more data to further improve your journey with diabetes. However, appropriate candidates should also have the following traits.

Willingness to Wear a Sensor
If you are going to start using a CGM, you need to know that you will have a sensor and a transmitter constantly attached to you. You might want to tape a transmitter to your skin to see what it is like to have a sensor.

A Good Support System
As with most aspects of diabetes, going it alone is not the best approach. Having your parents, family members, spouse, and friends involved can help you learn how and where to insert sensors, how to troubleshoot problems, and how to best use the information generated by the CGM. With support, your likelihood of success increases.

A Diabetes Team Familiar with CGM
You need a knowledgeable and accessible diabetes team that is experienced in teaching people how to get the best outcomes with a CGM.

Willingness to Change
The information obtained with CGM might indicate that you need to make significant changes to your diabetes regimen. You must be open to these changes to make CGM worthwhile.

Enough Body Fat to Wear a Sensor

Everyone has enough fat, but for young children and those who are very thin, these body areas might be somewhat limited for both a CGM and an insulin pump.

Skin That Can Tolerate CGM

You will need to use adhesive to secure the sensor and the transmitter. It might take some time to find the best way to secure the devices and give the body areas you use time to heal between insertions.

Cost of CGM

Health insurance coverage and the cost of a CGM must be taken into consideration. If your insurance does cover CGM, you still might have a large co-pay. You should be sure that you are able to bear the cost of a CGM before you decide to purchase and use one.

CHAPTER REVIEW

➡ Use a CGM if you want the extra information the glucose sensor provides. It gives hundreds of glucose values per day, alerts you if glucose values are outside your target range or are changing rapidly, shows trend graphs, and can upload data to computer programs for later analysis. For a CGM to help improve diabetes care, you need to know what to do with all the additional information and how to use it in collaboration with your diabetes team.

➡ There are many common misconceptions about CGM. You must understand that CGM does not replace SMBG, that it gives a lot of information, and that the simultaneous values for CGM and SMBG might be different because of the different conditions under which the glucose levels are measured.

➡ CGM should be considered if you experience wide fluctuations in glucose levels; have frequent, severe, unrecognized, or nocturnal hypoglycemia; have trouble with glucose control during exercise or periods of stress; have not achieved your target A1C; or want more information for your journey with diabetes.

CHAPTER 15

HOW TO USE CONTINUOUS GLUCOSE MONITORS AND PUMPS

There are a few different CGM systems available in the U.S. market. You should discuss which system you want with your diabetes team and with friends who are already using a CGM. Do your research too. Visit the CGM manufacturer websites. You might also want to go to the websites of diabetes associations and groups to see if they have any recommendations. Like everything with diabetes, you need to have information in order to make the right choice for you.

The major differences among different CGM devices are in the size and insertion angle of the sensors, how long the sensors last, whether the monitor is separate or integrated with an insulin pump, the look and feel of the sensor inserter, how often the CGM needs to be calibrated, what alerts are available, and what is displayed on the monitor with regard to arrows, trend graphs, and other numbers.

CGM DATA AND WHAT IT MEANS

The receiver gives you a ton of information and alerts. You must know how to use this information and those alerts in order to benefit from the information.

> **ALWAYS USE SMBG**
>
> Do not treat yourself based solely on information from the CGM. If you notice something that needs to be addressed, check your blood glucose first to help guide your actions.

Trend Arrows

All CGMs show trend arrows. Trend arrows tell you if your glucose levels are stable, rising or falling moderately (1–2 mg/dL a minute), or rising or falling quickly (more than 2 mg/dL a minute). Different systems have different designs for these arrows, but they all essentially display the same information: the rate of change of glucose levels and the direction in which they are going.

Trend arrows can be used to adjust your diabetes management plan. When combined with the current glucose value shown on a CGM, trend arrows will give you a forecast of your glucose levels, just like a weather forecast. If your current level is within your target range but the trend arrows indicate that your levels are rising or falling rapidly, you will know to take action now to prevent anything from actually happening, be that action issuing a correction bolus from your pump (for highs) or taking some glucose tabs or adjusting your basal rate (for lows). Similarly, if you are about to eat and your glucose level is in the target range but you have two arrows going up, you might consider increasing your meal insulin dosage (after you check your blood glucose level) or increasing the time between taking your bolus and starting your meal.

CORRECTING WITH TREND ARROWS

You can use trend arrows to correct a glucose value out of your target range. If you have one arrow going up and you need to take a correction dose of insulin for a high glucose value (confirmed with SMBG), then you add 10% more to the correction. If there are two arrows going up, add 20% more. If you are going to take a correction and you have one arrow going down, decrease by 10%, and for two arrows, decrease by 20%.

↑	↑↑	↓	↓↓
+10%	+20%	−10%	−20%

Alarms and Alerts

Alarms and alerts add tremendous value, but they must be set correctly. If the alarms and alerts are not set correctly, you may have alarms going off all the time, which will make you eventually so used to hearing them that you don't pay attention to them or even notice them (this is called alarm fatigue). Moreover, your alarms and alerts will change from your initial settings as you gain more experience using a CGM.

Alarms and alerts help with the early detection of glucose values heading out of the target range. They can warn you when you are about to go out of the target range (these are called predictive alerts) or when glucose values are changing rapidly (these are called rate-of-change alerts). They are especially valuable if you have trouble recognizing low glucose (this is called hypoglycemia unawareness), rapidly falling glucose levels, or concerns about hyperglycemia.

Most alarms can be programmed, so you can set your high and low glucose thresholds, how early you want the predictive alarm to go off (generally 20 or 30 minutes before you reach a specified value), and if you want the alarms to repeat. All alarms take several buttons or keystrokes to disable, ensuring that they are not accidentally turned off and that you notice the alarm. Alarms can be set at different volumes, so nighttime alarms can wake you up and daytime alarms won't interrupt classes or the workplace. These are all of the alarms that are available for the CGM.

- Threshold alarms: high or low glucose level reached.

- Predictive high and low alarms: about to go out of target range.

- Rate-of-change alarms: levels are rising or falling rapidly.

- Low-battery (receiver or transmitter) alarm: battery will need to be recharged or replaced.

- Lost sensor alarm: the CGM has lost the signal from the sensor and transmitter.

- Weak signal alarm: the CGM is not receiving a strong signal from the sensor and transmitter.

Low-Glucose Threshold Alarm

When you first begin using a CGM, you may want to set only the low-glucose threshold alarm. You may want to set it at a relatively low value, until you get used to CGM and alarms. As you become more experienced, you will want to increase this threshold, so you can help keep your glucose levels under tighter control.

High-Glucose Threshold Alarm

You might not want to set a high glucose threshold alarm when you first start using a CGM. As you gain experience and as your glucose levels improve, you may set this threshold rather high—around 300 mg/dL or so—and then gradually decrease it to help prevent highs. Eventually, you might want this alarm set at the upper level for your target range to better manage your glucose levels.

Predictive High and Low Alarms

You should not set these at the beginning of CGM use. These predictive high and low alarms should be set once you have your threshold alarms at the levels that work best for you.

Set the predictive alarm to notify you if you are going to reach your high or low threshold in 10 minutes. Once you get used to responding to this alarm and succeed in using it to prevent highs and lows, you might want to increase the time frame to 15 or 20 minutes. With predictive alarms, you have to get used to the fact that they might go off when your glucose level is still normal but on its way out of your target range. You can administer a small bolus to avert rising glucose levels or take a small amount of carbohydrate to prevent going low. After treating, view your trend graph and trend arrows to be sure that you are averting hitting the threshold. If not, the threshold alarm will sound.

Rate-of-Change Alarm

This is the last alarm you will set on the CGM. Wait until you are familiar with all of the other alarms and they are at their optimal settings. The rate-of-change alarm goes off when your glucose is trending up or down at a rapid rate. It may go off when your glucose level is in your target range. When rate-of-change alarms are used successfully, they can help you completely avoid highs and lows by giving you enough warning to treat your glucose when it is trending high (take a small correction bolus or temporarily increase your basal rate) or trending low (comsume extra carbohydrate or temporarily decrease your basal rate).

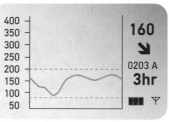

3-Hour Glucose Trend Graph

Graphs

You can view graphs of your glucose levels (sensor glucose on the y-axis, vertically, and time on the x-axis, horizontally) on your CGM. Graphs display your sensor glucose levels over various time periods: 3, 6, 12, and 24 hours. The display indicates your target range, so you can see if the CGM readings are in your target range.

CGM's have companion software that you can use to review several days' worth of information on your computer. The receiver stores the information, even though you cannot see it on the monitor itself. Learning how to review this information is essential to improving your glucose control.

Current Value

Your current sensor glucose value is displayed on the home or first screen that comes up when you activate the monitor. This screen updates every one to five minutes.

WHAT'S INVOLVED WITH WEARING A CGM

There are some daily maintenance tasks that you will need to do to ensure that your sensor is functioning properly and staying in place. As with an insulin pump, doing a quick assessment of your sensor every day will help prevent sudden problems and lower the odds of you having to do a lot of troubleshooting.

Inserting the Sensor

Begin by prepping your skin, loading the injector, applying any topical adhesive aids, inserting the sensor, and covering the area with tape afterward. Put the CGM in place, tell the receiver that you have inserted a new sensor, and wait for it to receive the signal from the new sensor. When it "finds" the new sensor, there is a warm-up period that will last 90–120 minutes. This warm-up period is needed to allow swelling to reduce at the site and wetting of the sensor.

After this warm-up period, the receiver will ask for a blood-glucose calibration from SMBG. For this calibration, you must test your blood glucose with a meter. The meter can be linked through radio frequency to the CGM, built into the monitor, or wholly separate. The receiver then uses algorithms (formulas) to calibrate the sensor according to the glucose reading from SMBG. This determines the glucose value that shows up on the CGM receiver screen. Each CGM device is slightly different, but most require calibration two times a day (or every 12 hours). But you may do more.

To successfully insert a sensor and have it stay in place for a long time (many CGM users have trouble with this), you must start with clean, dry skin. Do not apply oils, lotions, or creamy soaps. Thoroughly clean the entire area with alcohol to remove any natural oils or residue. If you are inserting the sensor in a place that has a lot of hair, you may want to consider shaving or trimming down the hair. If you perspire a lot, an unscented spray or solid antiperspirant can help. Apply the antiperspirant a couple of hours before inserting to allow the antiperspirant to work, then wipe the area with an alcohol swab. Some people like to use tape underneath or other solvent adhesive aids (these are products that can be used for pump sites too). It is not recommended to insert the sensor itself through tape, so if you need tape, cut a small hole in it where you plan to insert the needle.

Each sensor and its associated injector have specific loading methods. Most injectors are spring-loaded. After the sensor is inserted and the needle has been removed, check the site for bleeding. Some bleeding is normal. If there is bleeding, dab it with the corner of a tissue or cloth until it stops. Do not attach the transmitter to the

> **REMEMBER!**
>
> Your sensor, transmitter, and receiver are all technology and can be fragile! Treat them with care, avoid putting them into places where they might get cracked or scratched (e.g., a purse or luggage), and try to avoid dropping them.

sensor until the bleeding has stopped—this could affect the accuracy of the device. Once the bleeding has stopped, attach the transmitter to the sensor. Some sensors require a waiting period between insertion and transmitter attachment.

The transmitter can technically only be worn by clipping it into the sensor, but it is highly recommended that you place more tape over the top. You don't want to lose the transmitter; it is expensive. Try different ways to secure it. You might have to experiment a lot to find the best way to attach and secure your CGM.

Once your sensor is attached and has been secured and calibrated, it will send real-time CGM data, which can be seen on the receiver. While you are wearing the sensor, you need to check how it is functioning and how you are reacting to it at periodic intervals. Check to be sure that it is securely attached, that the batteries of the transmitter and receiver are charged and working, and that your skin is healthy (not red and no swelling). Remember, it is critical to calibrate the sensor with an SMBG reading two times a day. Try to calibrate before you go to bed, so you can avoid waking up to a calibration alarm or a nonfunctioning sensor if you sleep through the alarm.

After three to six or seven days, the sensor will expire. Remove the sensor and transmitter, recharge the batteries (if necessary), and take care of your skin—you will likely need that spot again soon.

You should note that if your sensor or transmitter falls off or comes out, then that sensor cannot be used. You cannot reinsert a used sensor. Once finished with your sensor, remove the transmitter and put the sensor part in your sharps disposal container. This is a good time to recharge your transmitter. If the battery on your transmitter goes out in the middle of a sensor's life, it can end the sensor's life as well. It's smart to always check battery life before you insert a new sensor so that you don't waste one because of a dead or low-charge battery.

Costs

The technology needed to run a CGM system with the three components is fairly advanced. The receiver is a one-time purchase, the transmitters need to be replaced about once or twice a year, and the sensors last only a few days.

On average, a CGM will cost you hundreds of dollars per month. Therefore, it is important for you to determine what you will have to pay for a CGM and what you are willing to pay. Call your insurance company and ask to speak to someone who is familiar with your plan's policy on diabetes supplies.

You must have a prescription for a CGM. Only you and your diabetes team can assess whether you (and your family) are ready for a CGM. Your team should also be able to help you choose which device will work best for you. They should help set up your training— either by training you themselves or by arranging a training session with a representative from the CGM manufacturer. Training takes from three to six hours. You should anticipate follow-up visits, calls, or e-mails to adjust alarms, to adjust your insulin regimen, and to discuss your treatment plan for highs and lows. Uploading and reviewing the data will help you and your diabetes team examine and understand your glucose levels, what is associated with highs and lows, and strategies to improve your diabetes management.

Getting a CGM can improve your diabetes control when the device is properly used and the data is effectively reviewed. By adjust-

NEW IN BOX

Start-up kits for CGM systems include the receiver/monitor, a transmitter, and several sensors.

ing your diabetes regimen in response to your glucose trends and patterns—and by using real-time values and alerts and alarms—you should be able to make your journey with diabetes the best and safest that it can possibly be.

CHAPTER REVIEW

➡ A CGM generates a lot of data. There are trend arrows, alarms, alerts, graphs, and the current sensor glucose value. Using CGM data effectively will allow you to get the best results out of your CGM and your diabetes management.

➡ There are some daily maintenance tasks you need to do to ensure that your sensor is functioning properly and staying in place. As with an insulin pump, do a quick assessment of your sensor every day to help prevent problems and reduce the amount of potential troubleshooting. You also need to know how to properly insert your sensor and ensure that it stays on.

➡ A CGM can improve your diabetes control when properly used and understood. By adjusting your diabetes regimen in response to the glucose trends and patterns provided by a CGM, and by taking advantage of real-time values and alerts and alarms, you should be able to make your journey with diabetes the best and safest that it can be.

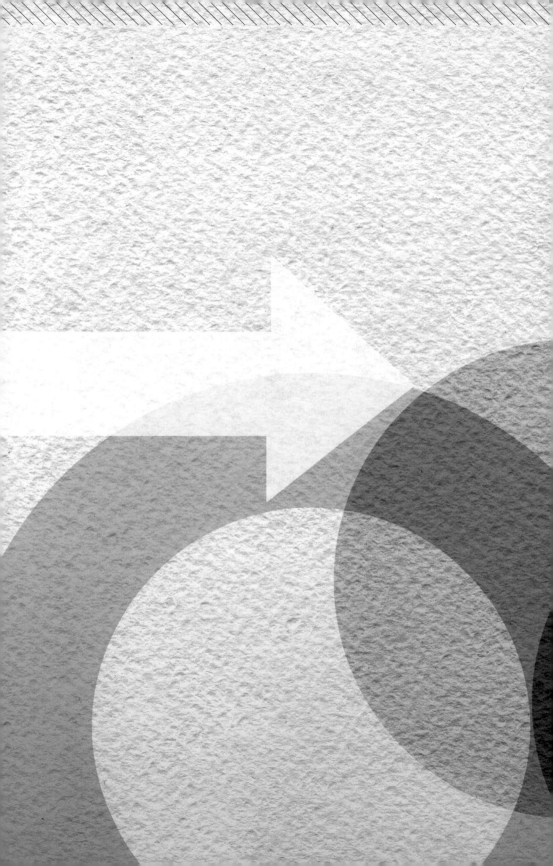

A LOOK INTO THE FUTURE

IN THIS CHAPTER

- The Components of the Artificial Pancreas
- The Steps to the Artificial Pancreas
- Conclusion

CHAPTER 16

A LOOK INTO THE FUTURE

Over the last 30 years, there have been remarkable advances in insulin pump therapy. Over the last 12 years, the same can be said for continuous glucose monitoring. These advances have enabled over a half million people around the world to benefit from using insulin pumps and hundreds of thousands of people from continuous glucose monitoring. But the ultimate promise has yet to be realized—fully automated insulin delivery with the artificial pancreas.

THE COMPONENTS OF THE ARTIFICIAL PANCREAS

The components of the artificial pancreas are the insulin pump, the continuous glucose sensor, and mathematical equations—called algorithms—that determine how much insulin should be given minute by minute. We call this system "closing the loop" because there is a "loop" that goes between the pump and sensor. That loop right now is open because a person has to take the sensor information and tell the pump what to do. "Closing the loop" means that information from the sensor will be used automatically in the algorithms to direct the minute-by-minute insulin delivery by the pump.

Although we know of the basic components of the artificial pancreas, there are a number of questions concerning how these components will function, what they need to offer, and how they need to be changed and put together. Much research needs to be done to develop a system that will deliver on the promise of the closed loop. Some of the key questions for an artificial pancreas follow.

What Is the Best Algorithm?

Closed-loop algorithms are being used now in a number of other closed-loop systems, such as the automatic pilot in planes, the thermostat in your house, and the cruise control in your car. A lot of research is being done to develop effective, safe algorithms that can be used in the artificial pancreas.

Is Delivering Only Insulin Sufficient?

Does the artificial pancreas truly have to mimic how the pancreas functions and also have the ability to give glucagon to prevent hypoglycemia? Would the system benefit from giving another hormone, such as pramlintide or a glucagon-like peptide-1 (GLP-1) analog, since both decrease after-meal glucose rises? Pramlintide (from the beta-cell) and GLP-1 (from the intestinal tract) are hormones that are currently used to treat diabetes, and it is possible that they may improve glucose management for people using the artificial pancreas. Conceptually, any of these other hormones might only need to be given intermittently (such as glucagon when the glucose level is falling or pramlintide when a meal is being ingested). Therefore a pump used in the artificial pancreas may require two chambers (one for insulin and one for the other hormone), or two separate pumps may be needed.

Is the Insulin Now Used Good Enough?

You know that your rapid-acting insulin still acts much more slowly than the insulin released from the pancreas. This is because there is still a delay in its absorption from your subcutaneous tissue, and its main site of action—your liver—is far away. Several strategies could accelerate insulin action to create an effective artificial pancreas. These include newer, more rapid-acting insulins; new developments in infusion sets; and delivering insulin into the abdominal cavity to get closer to the liver.

Is One Sensor Good Enough?

Because the sensor is critical in determining how much insulin needs to be given minute by minute, the artificial pancreas might require two sensors. With two sensors, the glucose readings must match for the artificial pancreas to continue to direct insulin delivery. If the glucose readings don't match, then the system could be redirected to give only preset basal insulin, like the insulin pump does now.

THE STEPS TO THE ARTIFICIAL PANCREAS

It is likely that the full artificial pancreas will be developed by incrementally adding automated features to the sensor-augmented pump system. The information from the sensor will control more and more of the insulin-delivery process before it controls the entire system. What are the potential incremental steps?

Low-Glucose Suspend
This feature allows for insulin delivery to be suspended when a predetermined glucose threshold is reached. For example, if you want to reduce the time you spend under 70 mg/dL, you set the low-glucose suspend to stop insulin delivery at 70 mg/dL.

Predictive Low-Glucose Suspend
This feature would allow insulin delivery to be suspended when the glucose level is predicted to hit 70 mg/dL in a predetermined amount of time, such as 15–30 minutes. This would help prevent low blood glucose altogether.

Treat to Range
This feature would allow for an automatic increase in basal insulin delivery or allow for an automatic bolus if there is a sustained high glucose level.

Closed Loop at Night
This would make the full closed loop—minute-to-minute automated insulin delivery—possible at night.

Full Closed Loop

The final step will be complete automation of insulin delivery in response to minute-by-minute glucose levels.

CONCLUSION

Over the last few decades, we have witnessed incredible advances in diabetes therapies: new rapid-acting insulins; smaller, faster glucose meters; information management with uploaded data from glucose monitors, pumps, and sensors; and next-generation pumps and sensors. We have come a long way, and the reality of an artificial pancreas is essentially within sight. The end result will be the near-perfect control of glucose levels without much human intervention. We owe thanks to the diabetes associations, including the American Diabetes Association (ADA), the Helmsley Trust, and the Juvenile Diabetes Research Foundation (JDRF); to the National Institutes of Health; and to many investigators and researchers around the world. But most importantly, we owe thanks to each of you. Those of you who strive to manage diabetes, who use advanced therapies and technologies to get the best results, and who wait for each step on the road to the artificial pancreas.

A BRIGHT FUTURE

Some call this the "closed-loop system" or an "artificial pancreas," but regardless of the terms used, a person with diabetes will, hopefully, eventually be able to receive the proper dose of insulin without even having to think about it—just like a person who doesn't have diabetes. With the promise of the artificial pancreas, the future is bright.

INDEX

ABOUT THE AUTHOR

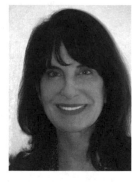

Francine R. Kaufman, MD, is a distinguished professor emerita of pediatrics and communications at the Keck School of Medicine and the Annenberg School of Communications at the University of Southern California. She was also the head of the Center for Endocrinology, Diabetes, and Metabolism at Children's Hospital Los Angeles until 2009, when she became the chief medical officer and VP of global clinical, medical, and health affairs for Medtronic Diabetes. In 2003, she was the president of the American Diabetes Association.